W9-BMO-710

Trials of
an Expert
Witness

Trials of an Expert Witness

TALES OF
CLINICAL NEUROLOGY
AND THE LAW

Harold L. Klawans, M.D.

Little, Brown and Company
BOSTON   TORONTO   LONDON

Library of Congress Cataloging-in-Publication Data

Klawans, Harold L.
    Trial of an expert witness: tales of clinical neurology and the
law / by Harold L. Klawans. — 1st ed.
        p.   cm.
    Includes index.
    ISBN 0-316-49683-9
    1. Forensic neurology — Anecdotes.   2. Forensic neuropsychology —
Anecdotes.   I. Title.
    RA1147.K56   1991
    614'.1 — dc20   90-6509

10 9 8 7 6 5 4 3 2 1

HC

Book design by Robert G. Lowe

Published simultaneously in Canada
by Little, Brown & Company (Canada) Limited

Printed in the United States of America

For Barbara
with love

Contents

Acknowledgments

Many individuals helped me to obtain and interpret the basic background materials required for these essays. Special thanks are due to Francis M. Forster and Harold Stevens, two neurologists whom I have known for well over twenty years. Each of them had personal involvement with one of the cases included in this book; Frank Forster was a witness in the Jack Ruby trial, while Harold Stevens was one of Ezra Pound's nontreating physicians. Both Frank and Harold discussed their experiences with me, and, most fortunately, each had written out his own reminiscences, which both were kind enough to allow me to read.

Numerous lawyers also assisted me. I have decided, however, not to name them. Although all of the court cases included here are public record, I have changed the names and other key details, including jurisdictions (locations), to protect the anonymity of the patients. Giving the names of the lawyers could compromise this principle.

Trials of
an Expert
Witness

CHAPTER ONE

The Rules of the Game

Winning isn't everything. It's the only thing.

— Vince Lombardi
Coach
Greenbay Packers

This is a court of law, young man, not a court of justice.

— Oliver Wendell Holmes
Chief Justice
United States Supreme Court

Jacques Barzun is credited with having proclaimed that "whoever would know the heart and mind of America had better learn baseball." While I will never dispute that axiom, the single action that has come to epitomize much of the American character to me belonged to a figure from an entirely different and much more international sport, namely, basketball. "Red" Auerbach was for many years the coach of the most successful basketball team in the world, the Boston Celtics, who won ten championships in a single eleven-year stretch under his leadership. He was an intense competitor who fought tooth and nail, but as soon as he knew that the game was won, Red relaxed, sat back, and lit a cigar, barely watching either his team or their opponents play out the rest of the game. That act was not one of disdain or arrogance. He had won. He had no more worries. He could relax and enjoy himself. He could sit back and feel the thrill of victory. If his actions increased the agony of defeat, so be it.

This approach to life is unknown to physicians and scientists. Yet I felt no loss in its absence. I could always turn on the TV and watch the Boston Celtics. But that all changed with Donna McKnight. She became my entrée into the arena of adversarial law, the battlefield of winning and losing. It was because of her that I first became an expert witness. On the day she first came into my office, I had no clear idea what constituted an expert witness or what an expert witness actually did. And like most other physicians, if given the choice, I would have rejected the idea of becoming involved with any legal processes. They were far too messy. And lawyers couldn't be trusted. So why get started?

That was 1974. I was Director of Neurology at Michael Reese Hospital, one of Chicago's largest private hospitals. Donna had just turned twenty-three. She came to see me because she needed a neurologist. Her lawyer hadn't sent her. She didn't even have a lawyer yet. She came to me because I was the only neurologist she knew. I had treated her uncle who had Parkinson's disease. I had helped him. So when her doctor suggested that she might need a neurologist, she remembered my name and decided to come to see me.

Donna had been in an accident on one of Chicago's elevated trains. Every night she took the El home from work. The accident had occurred one evening between Christmas and New Year's Eve. The El train she was riding home in was stopped at a station, waiting. It had been there for ten minutes, not an unusual occurrence in Chicago. Suddenly a second elevated train smashed into her train from behind. The second train had been slowing down to stop at the station, but it was still going along at a good clip. As always, Donna had been sitting in the back car, which was closest to the back stairs of her station. Donna heard the screech of metal against metal as the second train slammed on its brakes. And then the entire car shuddered. She was suddenly thrown forward. Her head almost flew off her neck.

Flexion of the neck, I thought to myself, as I listened to her recite her story.

Her head then snapped back as she saw the windows explode.

Followed by rapid extension. "Flexion-extension injury," I wrote in her chart.

The lights went out. People screamed. They cried. They moaned.

Donna checked herself. She was surprised; she felt fine. No blood anywhere. No cuts. No broken bones, as far as she could tell. The paramedics arrived within minutes. She told them she was fine. Other people were in far worse shape. Still, they took her to the nearest E.R. There she was seen by a doctor who spoke hardly any English. He talked to her for thirty seconds, examined her for another thirty, and ordered all sorts of X rays of her head and shoulders. He then sent her home with a diagnosis of whiplash and concussion, a prescription for a mild muscle relaxant, and a bill for $190. She never bothered to get the prescription filled. She felt fit as a fiddle. Within hours all that changed.

Her neck started to hurt. The E.R. doctor had mentioned something about a possible whiplash. She assumed that a little neck pain was to be expected. It was nothing to worry about. Her neck pain was mild at first. But in a short time, it became more than mild. More intense. Sharper. And her neck got stiff. It hurt to move her neck even a little bit. But it wasn't the neck pain that worried her. Or the stiffness. She was having trouble walking. She walked as if she were drunk. She couldn't understand that. She'd known lots of people who had been in accidents and had whiplash injuries. None of them had walked as if they were drunk.

Or had they at first?

She didn't really know.

So Donna went to bed to see if a good night's sleep would help. It didn't. The next morning she still walked as if she were drunk.

And it still hurt to move her head. Getting out of bed was torture. Perhaps God was telling her something. Stay in bed. So Donna stayed home from work the next day. That didn't help, either. In fact, after a couple of hours in bed, she started having trouble seeing.

She wanted to call a doctor, but, like many other women her age, her only physician was her gynecologist, and although she used him for many things aside from her annual pelvic examination, Donna knew that he was not the right doctor for this problem. She was having double vision, and she was walking as if she were drunk. And it had all started with that accident she'd had on the El just the day before.

She had no other choice. She called her doctor. He was on vacation. The nurse suggested that she go to the E.R. She'd already done that once.

The nurse then suggested bed rest.

She tried that. It hadn't helped.

Perhaps she needed a neurologist.

Donna agreed and then remembered my name, called my office, and became my patient.

I took the rest of her history. Prior to the elevated-train accident, she'd never had a neurological symptom. Now she had two: a drunken gait and double vision.

I examined her. The exam confirmed that she had the two separate problems she had complained about: a drunken gait and double vision. I didn't use those terms; I called them ataxia and diplopia, since those are the words neurologists use. Ataxia is a specific form of gait imbalance due to altered or abnormal function of the cerebellum or the tracks leading to or from it. Donna had something wrong with her cerebellum or its connections. Diplopia, or double vision, means that the two eyes are not simultaneously focusing on precisely the same place. It implies an abnormality in the brain stem in those areas in the back of the brain that control eye movement. Donna also had one other, more minor, problem. She didn't even know it. She had sensory loss in both feet. Up to her ankles. Her ability to appreciate vibration — specifically, the vibrations of a tuning fork — was markedly reduced. That loss implied an abnormality in the pathway carrying vibratory sensation to her brain. Almost always that means a problem in the spinal cord.

Three problems in three separate neurological systems:

Cerebellar.

Brain stem.

Spinal cord.

Multiple problems that could not come from a single spot in the nervous system. To a neurologist, what she had resembled a first episode of multiple sclerosis.

At that time, the diagnosis of M.S. was based entirely on clinical grounds. There were no really reliable biochemical tests. Patients were diagnosed as having M.S. if their disease included multiple areas of involvement of the brain and spinal cord, separate in space and time. Donna only fulfilled one half of the definition. She had multiple areas of involvement scattered in space — three different parts of her nervous system weren't working right. But this was her first episode. There was no scattering over time. Her symptoms had all started close together, within twenty-four hours. That made them part of a single attack. M.S. is characterized by recurring episodes. Perhaps she would never have another one.

Today, we can do far more sophisticated testing. One of these is the NMR or MRI — magnetic imaging of the brain and spinal cord, which can often demonstrate the multiple lesions themselves. The abnormal areas can now be seen, not inferred. There are tests of various kinds of evoked potentials. These are physiologic tests that show how electrical impulses are carried to the brain and can pinpoint where the nerve tracts are injured. And there are also more specific tests of the immune system. We don't really know what M.S. is or what causes it, but we do know that part of the process involves the production and appearance of abnormal antibodies in the injured areas of the nervous system. The presence of these antibodies can be detected in the spinal fluid. These are not definitive tests for the disease, but if a patient lacks the antibodies, it is quite unlikely that that patient has true M.S.

Back in 1974, we had no MRI. The CT scan had just been invented. No one was quite sure how accurate or helpful evoked potentials were. And all we could measure in the spinal fluid was the total amount of immune protein — the amount of gamma globulin. We couldn't characterize it. Most of the workup then consisted of proving that the patient didn't have any other disease.

So I admitted Donna to the hospital and started out trying to prove what she didn't have. We did a CT scan. It was normal. No brain tumor. No abnormal blood vessels in the brain. We did a spinal tap. No evidence of infection. The gamma globulin was slightly increased. We did lots of blood tests to rule out other diseases. They all came back normal.

So what did she have?

In all probability, M.S. But only one attack. A puzzlement. What do you tell a patient? She might not have M.S. And even if she did, she might not have another attack for fifteen or twenty years. Would it be fair to give her the label of M.S.?

"What do I have?" she asked.

"Areas of inflammation in your brain and spinal cord," I said.

"You mean M.S.?"

She was very smart.

"Perhaps, but we're not certain."

I placed her on steroids to decrease the inflammation. She started to improve; but the day before she was scheduled to go home, all that changed. Her double vision was gone. Her walking was ever so slightly improved. Then she woke up and couldn't see anything out of her right eye. That answered the question. She had now had a second episode separated in time. She now had multiple areas separated in space and time. So much for euphemisms. Donna had multiple sclerosis. I knew it and she knew it.

I prescribed more steroids. And once again, this was followed by partial improvement. The vision in her right eye improved about 80 percent.

I followed her as an outpatient. For the next six months, nothing happened. Her walking was still quite unsteady. Her vision in her right eye was slightly impaired. There was no double vision, and her vibratory sensation was all but back to normal. She had never known it was decreased.

Despite the improvements, she had all she could do to get to work. She couldn't ride the El anymore. The steps were too hard to navigate, especially if it rained and they got slippery. She dreaded winter and the ice and snow.

And she was worried about her next attack. Now it was no longer *if*. It was *when*.

I tried to reassure her. It might never come. It might be years away.

But it could be tomorrow, she reminded me.

I couldn't refute that. Only time would define her course.

And time was not easy on her. She spent most of it waiting for her next attack.

Her lawyer called me. The Chicago Transit Authority wanted to settle her claim. Her medical bills were $190 for the E.R. visit and $100 for my initial evaluation. A total of $290. They were offering her $2,900. Not bad. He was going to tell her to take it.

"Unless the accident brought on her M.S.," I mused offhandedly.

"Can accidents do that?" he asked hopefully.

"I'm not sure. But there is an entire medical literature on the subject."

"There is?"

I could imagine the dollar signs in his eyes.

"There is."

"Who knows that literature?"

"I do."

"Would you like to be Donna's expert?"

As optimistic as I tried to be with Donna, I knew she would have other attacks. She would develop increased disability over the years. The odds were stacked against her. I wanted to help her.

Money couldn't buy her a normal nervous system, but as my mother had once so wisely said, "There's no problem that having more money aggravates."

But did I really believe that trauma could precipitate M.S.? I wasn't certain.

I also wasn't certain what an expert witness was and what he did. Marshall Goldberg knew and he explained it all to me.

I was Donna's doctor. In legal terms, that meant that I was a "subsequent treating physician." She had come to me for treatment and I had voluntarily agreed to undertake her care.

I had, I readily admitted.

I could be subpoenaed to give evidence.

I could?

Yes.

And I had no choice?

None. I was her treating physician.

Did I have to give an opinion?

No, he grudgingly admitted.

Not opinions. Just the facts. I could be subpoenaed to give evidence as to what had happened — like any other witness. And since I was a subsequent treating physician, it would be assumed that what she told me had been true.

"What does an expert do?"

"He gives an opinion."

"Such as?"

"That the accident caused the M.S."

"Not caused, brought on."

"Whatever."

"As a subsequent treating physician, can't I do that?"

"You can, but . . ." He stopped.

"But what?"

"An expert gets paid for his time. A treating physician has no choice. He has to testify. An expert bills for his time."

"What defines an expert?"

"Acknowledged expertise. Are you board certified in neurology?"

"Of course. I'm head of neurology here. I'm a full professor of neurology at the University of Chicago. I've published over seventy papers on neurology."

"You're an expert." He paused. "You're hired."

"You don't even know my opinion."

"Is it your opinion to the best of your medical judgment that the accident could or might have caused Donna McKnight's M.S.?"

"Precipitated," I corrected him.

"Whichever."

"Yes."

"Is that more probably than not?"

"More probably than not could have precipitated the M.S.?" I inquired, rewording the complete question.

"Yes," he replied anxiously.

"I suppose so. I'd have to reread the literature. But I don't believe that it did beyond the benefit of a doubt."

"Beyond the benefit of a doubt doesn't apply. That's for criminal law. This is civil law. All we have to prove is 'more probably than not.' Fifty-one percent to forty-nine percent. That's all. Not ninety-nine. Just that, in your opinion, it's more probably than not."

"What if I don't really believe that it's been proved scientifically?"

"I don't care what you believe to be proved as an absolute scientific fact. This is a game we play. And like every other game, this game has its own set of rules. We need an expert. You qualify as an expert. The expert, based on the facts of the case and his expert knowledge of the medical literature and his experience, reaches an opinion. Not an absolute opinion. Not scientific proof to be published in the *New England Journal of Medicine*. An opinion which is more probably true than not."

"More probably than not."

"That's it. It's the other side's job to get an expert who has a different opinion, and then it's up to the jury to decide. And juries like sick patients better than they like the Chicago Transit Authority. It's all one big game, Doc. And like any other game, you play to win."

Winning was not the issue, I said to myself. Telling the truth was. That and helping Donna. Winning one for Donna.

I told him I'd review the literature and we'd talk again.

"How much does an expert witness get?" I asked.

"Fifty an hour," he mumbled.

"Including the time I spend reviewing the literature?"

"Yes," he admitted grudgingly.

"No matter what happens?"

"If you're engaged to be an expert, you get paid the same whether your side wins or loses. That's the law. You can't have an economic stake in winning."

"What happens if I review everything and decide it's no go?"

"You'll still get paid. You're paid for your time. Not your opinion."

That's how we left it.

I reviewed the literature, and two weeks later Marshall Goldberg came by my office to discuss the case with me. The literature supported the possible relationship between trauma and the precipitation of an attack of M.S.

"Don't ever say that," he admonished me.

"Say what?"

"Possible. Possible has no legal meaning. Anything is possible. It's got to be probable or it's nothing. And probable . . ."

"I know," I interrupted him, "means more probably than not. Fifty-one percent."

"Well?"

"It's a go," I said, and began to reel off the articles I had read.

"Save that for court," he said. "I don't need facts. Just your opinion."

I was to be his expert. He would file his case, *McKnight v. CTA*. First, I would have to supply a letter outlining my opinion. Then I would have to give "an evidentiary deposition." That was so the other side could discover what my opinions were. Then if the case wasn't settled without a trial, I would have to testify in court.

My court appearance took place some two years later. Goldberg and I met the day before I was to testify. I wanted him to understand my testimony. All he wanted was a list of questions he should ask me.

I gave them to him.

"Now let me tell you how to talk to a jury."

I stopped him. "That I know."

"How do you know that?"

"I'm a teacher," I said. "That's what I do for a living. I teach medical students. So, I'll teach the jury. Twelve jurists in a courtroom can't be too different from a dozen students at a bedside. You teach them one at a time. You look from one to the other, maintaining eye contact, making sure they understand, going back and forth. That keeps them all involved and interested. That I know how to do."

He was not entirely convinced, but I was not interested in his coaching. He talked about what I should wear. My clothes should be conservative, but not too expensive. A dark suit. Nothing flashy.

I showed up in a blue blazer with gray trousers and a conservative tie. I didn't own a dark suit. And I wasn't going to buy one just for appearance in court.

Since I was a witness for the plaintiff, Goldberg led me through my direct testimony. First, he had to qualify me as an expert in neurology. That was easy. It was done step-by-step.

Undergraduate education.

Medical school.

Internship.

Residency.

Board certification.

Academic appointments past and present, culminating in my appointment as a full professor at the University of Chicago.

My publications, including all the papers I had written and all the books I had written or edited.

These accomplishments meant that I was qualified to be considered an expert on neurological disease.

The defense conceded that point.

Then we moved on to Donna McKnight.

She was my patient, I told the court.

Her diagnosis?

Multiple sclerosis.

Could I explain what M.S. was.

I could. And I did. Not to Marshall Goldberg. He didn't care. Not to the judge. To the jury. Looking at them one at a time, answering their puzzled looks whenever possible, returning their nods, responding to each and every cue.

I talked about the diagnosis of M.S. — multiple areas of involvement of the brain and spinal cord separated by time and space. I talked about Donna McKnight and the evidence of multiple areas of involvement of her brain and spinal cord separated by time and space.

I talked about her disability.

I talked about her prognosis of increased disability.

Did we know the cause of M.S.?

No.

Did we know any factors that might bring about an attack of M.S. in a patient with known M.S.?

Yes.

Such as?

"Trauma," I said. "A bodily injury."

What was the basis of that opinion?

Back to the jury. I took a deep breath and looked at the heavyset black woman who was seated in the front row, closest to me. She was, I assumed, the foreman. Or forewoman. Foreperson. She smiled toward me and off I went.

"According to most authorities," I began, "an injury can be considered to have brought on M.S. if someone who was previously free of any clinical evidence of M.S. develops signs and symptoms of M.S. within a reasonable period following an injury."

Was that just my opinion? Goldberg inquired.

No.

Who else's?

"McAlpine. He's the author of the standard textbook on M.S. Doctor McAlpine believes that three separate factors have to be considered before deciding in any single patient whether or not a specific episode of trauma brought on the M.S. The first of these is the character, degree, and site of the trauma. The second is the time relationship between the injury and the appearance of the first symptoms of multiple sclerosis. And third is any evidence that suggests a relationship between the site of the injury and that of the initial symptoms. McAlpine believes that the time between the trauma and exacerbation of the disease should be short. Most authorities, including McAlpine and Russell, consider that the time period should be less than three months." By now, I was on a roll. The jury was with me, listening to my detailed explanation. And the defense was allowing me to do what I do best, lead. "As early as 1922," I continued, "the Association for Research in Nervous and Mental Disease concluded that some cases of multiple sclerosis were initiated by trauma. Trauma cannot itself cause it but may awaken the disease process," I added.

Had I relied on any other studies? Goldberg asked me. He read questions well. He was following the script I had given him. It was almost as if he were listening to what I was saying.

"The study of McAlpine and Compston was published by the *Quarterly Journal of Medicine* in 1952. That's the most complete study of the relationship of trauma to multiple sclerosis," I replied. "In this study, there was a history of trauma within three months of the onset of the initial symptoms in almost one-seventh of the patients. In most of these there was a correlation between the site of injury and the site of the initial lesion within the central nervous system. As a result of this study, McAlpine concluded that there was little doubt that trauma to a limb or any part of the body, slight or severe, might occasionally precipitate the disease in a predisposed person or might cause a relapse." I paused and surveyed the jury. They were still with me. "There is one other important study by Brain and Wilkinson. They found that trauma was often related to an exacerbation of multiple sclerosis, especially if the trauma involved the neck. All in all," I concluded, "the evidence from the medical literature on the relationship of trauma to multiple sclerosis suggests that trauma may have a relationship to the onset of multiple sclerosis in an individual if a trauma precedes the onset of signs and symptoms by less than three months. The shorter the period of time, the more likely the relationship."

Did Ms. McKnight have any signs or symptoms of M.S. prior to the accident?

No.

In my opinion, could trauma bring on M.S.?

Yes.

Was that opinion more probable than not?

Yes.

Was that opinion based upon my knowledge of the medical literature and my own experience?

Yes.

Did Ms. McKnight have M.S.?

Yes. More probably than not.

Did the El accident precipitate her attack of M.S.?

Yes.

That was the end of direct questioning. It was time for cross-examination.

"My name is James Duffy," the lawyer said. He was about sixty. I'd never met him before. He was a senior partner in a prominent Chicago firm that was connected well enough politically to represent the CTA. James Duffy wore a suit that must have cost six hundred dollars. He didn't waste his time at depositions. His firm had sent a young lawyer to take my deposition. Duffy's job was to destroy me in front of the jury. And he was supposed to be good at that. He was a street fighter who knew all the tricks of the trade.

Goldberg was also a street fighter. Not as well connected politically, but he, too, knew his way around the courtroom. He had warned me about impeachment. Impeachment is the standard way of demonstrating that an expert's testimony should not be believed. It can be done in one of two ways. The first is to show that a recognized authority, one the expert acknowledges to be a reliable authority, contradicts the expert's testimony. The second, and tougher, is to prove that the expert has contradicted himself. This is usually done by comparing statements the expert has previously made in the depositions in the case at hand, or testimony or depositions he has given in other cases.

Goldberg was certain that Duffy would try to impeach me. Getting another expert to contradict me would not be enough. I was not only an expert, I was also Donna's doctor. The defense expert was an outsider, so it was not just two hired guns shooting it out at the corral. And the jury would also tend to side with a passenger over the CTA. Duffy had to attack me.

But how?

Not by attacking my testimony. But by the use of authority.

Goldberg felt that the best defense was to say that I didn't recognize the authority of whatever book or article he brought up. If I said I didn't believe it was authoritative, it made no difference what the book said. I was prepared.

Duffy didn't beat around the bush. "Are you familiar with a *Textbook of Neurology* written by Dr. Baker?" he began.

Of course I was. Dr. Baker had trained me. I had read those four volumes from cover to cover — more than once. But Abe had not written them. He had been the editor, not the author. It was a multiauthored text, with more than forty authors involved. I debated saying that but opted to bide my time. "Yes," I replied.

Goldberg was getting nervous. He started to squirm in his chair. He had warned me. I shouldn't have said yes.

"And you are familiar with the chapter in this book on multiple sclerosis?" Duffy continued.

"Yes, sir," I replied, knowing instinctively that an expert should always be polite. But what was he getting at? The chapter had been written by a neurologist named Schumacher, from Vermont. It was one of my least favorite chapters in the entire set. Most of it was taken up with a long, cumbersome classification of diseases that were so rare that no patients ever had them. And no neurologist ever saw them.

"So you know this chapter?"

"I already said that." I knew that I didn't have to answer questions I had already answered once, but I did anyway. Goldberg was beyond squirming. He was very uncomfortable. And sweating.

"And Dr. Baker was your teacher, wasn't he?" Duffy was coming in for the kill — he had read my C.V. Goldberg was cringing.

"Oh, yes, sir."

"And this is an authoritative text, isn't it? In your opinion?"

He had asked the right question. If I said no, then he could not use the text to impeach since I did not recognize it as authoritative. But how could I say no to Baker's *Textbook?* Baker had trained me. It was obvious that Schumacher had said something that contradicted my opinion. And Duffy had managed to ask the question in the best way. He had asked me about the entire book — all four volumes — not the one chapter. Was Baker's book authoritative, not Schumacher's chapter? "Yes," I answered.

Goldberg was dying.

"Well, then, how do you explain what Dr. Baker wrote in his chapter on multiple sclerosis, sir? And he was your teacher, wasn't he?" With that, Duffy opened the book in order to read something to me.

"Dr. Baker did not write a single word about M.S. in his entire life," I said firmly.

"There is an entire chapter on M.S. in this book, isn't there?" he said just as firmly, but with a tinge of anger.

"Yes, sir." Ever so politely.

"And in that chapter, Dr. Baker, your teacher, wrote . . ."

"Dr. Baker did not write about M.S. in that book."

"He didn't?" Disbelief.

"No, sir."

Goldberg was ready to be buried. He could see the money flying out the window. His money. Even Donna's money.

"Not a chapter?" Duffy asked with a smile.

"Not a word. Not a sentence."

"Judge," Duffy said, looking at the jury for the first time, "I want this chapter written by Dr. Baker to be marked as a defense exhibit. This witness has just impeached himself."

"Dr. Baker did not write the chapter on M.S.," I said, interrupting Duffy's motion. "If you will please read the book which you have in your possession, Mr. Duffy."

"This book that Dr. Baker wrote?"

"Dr. Baker did not write that book. He merely edited it. The chapter on M.S. was not written by Dr. Baker. It was written by Dr. George Schumacher, of Vermont, who was never my teacher at all."

"Oh."

"And whose expertise I do not recognize."

"Do you still want that book marked as an exhibit?" the judge asked.

"No, sir," Duffy replied, not knowing quite where to go next.

Goldberg was no longer dying. He had been resurrected. As had his unimpeached witness. And much more. I had just made his opposition look foolish to the judge and, more importantly, to the jury. In essence, the case was over. The defense lawyer couldn't touch me. The case was won, decided not by the facts, but by the playing of the game. "I think I want that marked, Judge," Goldberg said.

"I don't think that that is necessary," the judge told him.

We had won. Had Goldberg been coaching the Celtics, he would have lit up a cigar. He had won.

When the jury brought back their verdict, Donna was awarded $280,000.

But I felt I had won. Not money, but a contest. A competition. A joust. I had gone to battle for an opinion and I'd won.

And it felt good. I, too, wanted to light up a cigar.

I had enjoyed the game far more than I had thought I ever would. I was smitten. I knew if asked I would play again. And besides, I got paid. Not much, but something. Fifty dollars an hour. That, I soon learned, was not the going rate. The average fee for an expert was about $125 per hour at the time. Goldberg had lied to me.

So what? We'd won. Donna had won. I had won. And winning was addicting. And I was hooked.

The CTA appealed the case. In the appeal, Duffy argued that there was no proof that M.S. could be caused by trauma. The jury had been wrong.

The appellate court upheld the decision.

We had won again.

The appellate court believed me. They said so in their opinion. It was a legal principle that they supported. The legal principle that in the absence of absolute scientific proof that trauma could cause M.S., an opinion that it could "more probably than not" was sufficient.

Duffy had never actually asked me about the passage in Baker's *Textbook*. I later looked it up. In his chapter, Schumacher decried the notion that trauma could cause or precipitate M.S. I would have had a hard time refuting a passage that Abe had allowed to be printed in his *Textbook*. There were other questions that I had not been asked that were far more critical. I had testified that more probably than not the accident had precipitated Donna's first attack of M.S. and caused her to have M.S. sooner than she would otherwise have had it. But how much sooner? I had instructed Goldberg not to ask me that. What he asked me was: "You mean she might not have had an attack for years?" My answer was "Yes." To have won, the defense only had to ask one series of questions:

"It is your testimony that the accident caused her to have an attack of M.S. sooner that she would have otherwise had it?"

"Yes."

"And that could have been years sooner?"

"Yes."

"Could it have been one decade sooner?"

"Yes."

"Could it have been just one year sooner?"

"Yes."

"Could it have been just one month sooner?"

"Yes."

"Could it have been just one week sooner?"

"Yes."

"Could it have been just one day sooner?"

"Yes."

"Could it have been just one hour sooner?"

"Yes."

"Could it have been just one minute sooner?"

"Yes."

"So it is possible that we are here merely because of one minute?"

"Yes."

Had Duffy even heard what I had said?

Was he unable to think fast enough?

Was the flaw in my argument not that apparent?

Two years later I found out that it was. I was on the El. I saw a woman. I recognized her, but who was she?

She smiled. Then I knew. She'd been the foreman of the jury. The foreperson.

She asked me if Ms. McKnight was still my patient.

She was.

She was glad they were able to give her some money. Poor woman. M.S. was a terrible disease. The CTA could afford it.

She'd been worried.

About what?

"That rich attorney never asked you the key question."

"What was that?"

"How much sooner?"

It had been apparent if you listened. She had. In my experience, juries usually do. More often than the lawyers. They're too busy doing other things.

I never worked with Marshall Goldberg again. His practice consisted primarily of minor personal injury cases. He couldn't afford an expert who expected an appropriate fee. Every once in a while he'd call for some free advice. And I'd give it to him.

Four or five years ago he was certain he finally had a case for me. *"McKnight Two,"* he called it. Another young woman with M.S. starting within days of an automobile accident.

An open-and-shut case.

She'd been normal.

Then whiplash.

Then M.S.

He would send me the records.

"Don't," I said.

"With a retainer," he added.

"No."

"One hundred an hour." By then the standard fee was two hundred per hour. At least he was consistent.

"Don't."

"Why not?"

"Minor trauma doesn't precipitate M.S."

"But in McKnight."

"I know what I said in McKnight. That was my opinion then. That was almost fifteen years ago. There's been more research since then. I don't have that same opinion today. Science moves forward."

"So it used to precipitate M.S. and it doesn't anymore?"

"That's about it." I tried to teach him about the newer research. He wasn't any more interested than he had been fifteen years earlier. Science was not his concern.

I found out a few months later that he had settled the case for $100,000. He had told the insurance company that he had discussed the case with me and he had sent them a copy of my testimony in the McKnight case.

They offered to settle.

He took the money and ran.

CHAPTER TWO

Locked In

A doctor's reputation is made by the number of eminent men
who die under his care.

— George Bernard Shaw

Bonnie Lawrence could not have been happier. She and Bill had
just celebrated their second wedding anniversary. And he couldn't
be sweeter. Or kinder. Or a better lover. She still blushed if she
thought too much about that. And everything was going well at
work for her and for Bill, too. Of course, he was the boss's son-
in-law. And she was pregnant. What could be better?

She could do with a little less morning sickness. In fact, she
could do with a lot less. It was something she would have to learn
to live with, her mother had told her. After all, she, too, had had
severe morning sickness — with all four of her pregnancies. And
she had had four healthy children, Bonnie and her three brothers.
And the morning sickness had kept her from putting on weight.
She still weighed exactly what she weighed the day she got married. Bonnie could not make that claim. She had gained ten pounds
in the past two years. Closer, in fact, to twelve.

Bonnie's morning sickness took care of all that. By the time she
had been pregnant for six weeks, she had lost eight pounds. And
her breasts had increased a whole cup size. From B to C. Bill
hadn't said anything, but Bonnie was certain he liked the change.
Too bad it wouldn't be permanent.

At eight weeks, she was down twelve pounds, and Bill was beginning to worry about her. She also looked pale. He insisted she see
an obstetrician. Not the G.P. who had delivered her and whom she
had gone to ever since she was born, but a real obstetrician. She
agreed. But which one? She asked her friends, and they all agreed.

John Greengrass was the busiest and the best. Bonnie liked the "best" part, but wasn't so sure she liked the "busiest." What if he was too busy to give her the attention she needed? What if he was too busy when the time came? When she really needed him?

Why couldn't she stay with old Doctor Westlake?

He was too old, her friends told her. John Greengrass was younger. And far handsomer. And she was too much of a worry-wart.

That she was. But she really had no idea why it mattered that Dr. Greengrass was handsome. Her best friend almost fell down, she laughed so hard.

"Trust me," she said. "It makes a difference. And besides, he is the best."

So she called Dr. Greengrass's office to make an appointment. He could see her the next day. The office was very nice. Three times as big as Dr. Westlake's. And the waiting room was not filled with kids with runny noses or measles or God knows what. Just other pregnant ladies and their husbands or mothers. She should have let Bill come with her. And there were great magazines to read. Filled with articles on pregnancy and what to do both before and after the baby comes. This was going to be fun. If only she would stop feeling nauseated.

And Dr. Greengrass was handsome. Very handsome. Six feet two or three. Broad shoulders. Narrow waist. Blond hair. And he didn't wear a white coat. He wrote a great sweater. Cashmere, she'd bet.

He took her history.

She'd lost too much weight, he said. He wanted to give her some medicine. And if she got any worse, she might have to go into the hospital for a while.

Why?

For intravenous feeding.

Then he examined her. He didn't even put on a white coat for that. She wasn't so certain she liked that. It was the most thorough exam she'd ever had. He even examined her breasts. Dr. Westlake had never done that. Then he put on gloves and examined the baby. He did it so quickly and smoothly she hardly felt it. He was good. The best. She smiled.

He gave her several prescriptions. Vitamins. Iron. Calcium. And something to stop her nausea and vomiting. She had to weigh herself every day. If she lost four more pounds, she'd have to go into the hospital.

He told her to come back in three weeks. That was on Friday.

On Sunday she weighed 110 pounds.

On Tuesday she weighed 108 pounds.

On Thursday she weighed 107 pounds.

On Saturday she weighed 107 pounds. She was holding her own. And she felt better.

On Monday she weighed 106 pounds.

She'd lost four pounds. The idea of going into the hospital frightened her. And she did feel better. She'd give it another day or two.

Tuesday: 106.

Wednesday: 107. She had been right. She was better.

But not for long.

Thursday: 105. She couldn't keep a thing down. She vomited time after time. All day long.

Friday: 104.

Saturday: 103.

Sunday: 102.

Eight pounds.

Bill called Dr. Greengrass.

Bonnie had to be admitted to the hospital.

When?

Immediately.

Was it an emergency? There was an office golf outing . . .

Yes. It was an emergency.

Bill drove her to the hospital. They got there just after noon. He thought that Dr. Greengrass would be there waiting for them.

"He's in the delivery room," the nurse told them. Her name was Pat Bell. She seemed very nice. She said that she'd call Dr. Greengrass for orders as soon as she got Bonnie into bed.

She weighed Bonnie: 99 pounds.

What had she weighed before she got pregnant? 120 or so.

"Twenty pounds," Nurse Bell clucked.

She took Bonnie's blood pressure: 80 over 55.

Did she know what her blood pressure usually ran?

"No. Why?"

"Too low," was all she said. "Now, into bed."

The nurse called the delivery room and talked to Dr. Greengrass. "Mrs. Lawrence," she said, "is hypotensive and dehydrated."

"BP?" he asked.

"Eighty over 55."

"She needs fluids. Let's give her a liter of 5 percent glucose and water every two hours until I get to see her. That'll be late this afternoon."

"Anything else?" the nurse asked.

"She should have nothing by mouth except maybe ice chips to suck on. I don't want her to vomit anymore."

The nurse started the IV and transcribed the order: 1,000 cc 5 percent glucose and water every two hours.

"Will she be okay?" Bill asked.

"Of course. Nothing can go wrong now," the nurse reassured him. "We'll give her fluids now. Sugar and water. That's what she needs. She hasn't had any food for days, and she's lost a lot of fluid."

"Dr. Greengrass . . ."

"He's in delivery. He'll be down as soon as he's done. He's right in the hospital."

"She is okay?"

"Yes. Why don't you go to your golf outing?"

He did just that. Bonnie insisted she felt better. She felt safe. Everything would be just fine.

The first bottle of glucose and water ran from twelve-thirty to two-thirty. Nurse Bell then started number two.

At three-thirty Nancy Merriman replaced Pat Bell. At four-thirty she started number three.

Bill got back at six. Had Greengrass seen her yet?

No.

Why not?

He was still in the delivery rooms.

Would the nurse call him?

She would. She did.

He would come as soon as he could. He had two women in labor and one might need a C-section.

"But . . ." Bill complained.

"Don't worry, darling," Bonnie said. "I already feel better. I haven't vomited once since I've been here. Six whole hours. I'm much better."

At six-thirty, Nancy Merriman started bottle number four. At eight-thirty, number five.

At nine, Bill went home. Bonnie told him to. She felt great. Wonderful. She wanted him to make love to her.

"In the hospital?"

"Yes."

He decided to go home.

Ten-thirty. Number five was in. Number six was started.

At eleven Nurse Grace Hatton replaced Nancy Merriman. She came in to see Bonnie.

How did Bonnie feel?

"I've got a headache," Bonnie said.

"Is it bad?"

"No."

At twelve, the nurse stopped by again. Bonnie was still awake. But she seemed very tired. And her voice was a little slurred.

"When did you last sleep?"

"Lass nighth."

Definitely slurred.

"How do you feel?

"Thuper. Wonderfulth."

"No headache?"

"No."

She debated calling Dr. Greengrass. She hated disturbing John at home. She called the delivery rooms. Maybe he hadn't left yet. He had. At eleven. He'd never seen Bonnie. He would probably see her first thing in the morning, at six or seven.

At twelve-thirty she started number seven. At one she went in to check Bonnie. Bonnie was asleep. In a very deep sleep. Grace gave her a nudge. Bonnie didn't move a muscle. A pinch brought on no more response.

"Poor girl," Grace thought to herself. "She must be exhausted."

At one thirty-five, as she was walking by Bonnie's room, Grace heard a cry, and then the bed started rattling. Grace ran into the room.

It wasn't the bed that was rattling. It was Bonnie. She was having a seizure. A convulsion. Her arms and legs were jerking back and forth. So was her head.

Grace knew enough not to try to force her mouth open or put anything in her mouth. In a few seconds the convulsion stopped.

She took Bonnie's vital signs as quickly as she could.

Pulse: 120. Fast but not too fast.

Blood pressure: 80/60. No change.

Pupils: Large. Equal. They reacted to light. They were normal.

Respirations: Deep. Slow. Regular.

Did she respond?

To touch? No.

To command? No.

To pain? No.

It was time to get help. She ran out to the nursing station and called for Dr. Greengrass. She remembered that he had left the delivery room. She called him at his home.

"What's up?" He yawned.

"It's Mrs. Lawrence."

"Who?"

"Your patient with hyperemesis gravidarum."

"Oh, Christ," he said, starting to wake up. "I forgot all about her. I had such a hectic day. How is she?"

"She's . . . sleeping."

"So should I be."

"Except, I can't wake her up. She had this sort of seizure and now I can't arouse her."

"What did you try?"

"Everything. Even pain by rubbing her sternum."

"You mean she's in a coma?"

"Yes," Grace Hatton admitted. She was an obstetrical nurse. She didn't throw around words like coma very often or very easily, but there was no denying that Bonnie Lawrence was, in fact, comatose. That was why she had called Dr. Greengrass in the first place.

Greengrass was now fully awake.

"She had a seizure and became comatose," the nurse said.

"How was she before the seizure?"

"Sleepy. No. Lethargic."

"It sure doesn't sound like an obstetrical problem. It's a medical problem. Call the E.R. doctor to see her, and call in an internist."

"Who?"

"Mac. John MacMillan. And," he continued, "make sure she's getting enough fluid."

"Yes, sir. Are you coming in?"

"What good could I do?" he replied.

Nurse Hatton hung up and then called the E.R. and Dr. Mac-Millan. As soon as they responded, she went back to Bonnie's room. The patient was lying in bed. Her breathing was hardly audible, but she was breathing. Slowly and shallowly.

Her pulse was slower: 80.

Her blood pressure was as low as it had been before. Greengrass was probably right. Bonnie needed more fluids. Grace opened the IV all the way. The rest of the bottle would be inside of her in less than ten minutes.

Grace called Bonnie by her name. There was no response. Shaking the bed, shaking Bonnie's shoulder, flashing a light in her eyes, rubbing her sternum, pinching her were all equally ineffective.

She was truly comatose.

Where were those doctors?

Right there.

It was the doctor from the E.R. Roy Temple. She told him what she knew.

Twenty-three years old.

Good health.

Pregnant.

Hyperemesis gravidarum.

Seizure.

Coma.

Pulse: 80.

BP: 80 over 50.

Respirations: slow and shallow.

"Not true," he said. "They're rapid and deep."

She listened. He was right. Her breathing had changed. But when?

"The IV's almost out," he said. "What is it?"

"Five percent glucose."

"Hang another," he told her.

She went out to get the bottle as Dr. Temple started to examine the patient. By the time she got back, Dr. Temple was already sitting down and writing some orders. She attached the next bottle. Bonnie was no longer breathing rapidly. Her respirations were once again slow and shallow.

"What do you think is wrong?" she asked.

"I'm not sure. Most likely she's had a sudden hemorrhage into her brain. That would explain the seizure."

"I see . . ." she replied.

"I want to get an EKG, and we'll get some routine blood tests. I'll draw the blood."

And he did. Grace called the lab to get someone to pick it up. Immediately.

The lab tech got there in two minutes. It took only another two minutes for Dr. Temple to get back with the EKG machine. He and Grace had started to attach the electrodes by the time John MacMillan got there.

Grace told him the same story that she had told Dr. Temple.

Twenty-three years old.

Good health.

Pregnant.

Hyperemesis gravidarum.

Seizure.

Coma.

Pulse: 80.

BP: 80 over 50.

Respirations: slow and shallow.

She hesitated and then amended her recitation. The respirations varied from slow and shallow to rapid and deep.

"How?"

She didn't know what to say. She didn't know how that happened. That was his job. He was the doctor.

"I don't know why."

"Not why, Ms. Hatton. How? Is the transition slow or all of a sudden?"

"I don't . . . No. Slow. One time she's breathing slowly and then fast, then slow, but the change isn't noticeable, so it must change slowly."

MacMillan nodded. He then examined Bonnie and stepped back while Roy Temple ran an EKG.

Together they read the tracing.

"Normal," MacMillan said.

"Normal," Temple agreed. "I think she's had a hemorrhage into her brain," he added.

MacMillan shook his head. "I doubt that. She's got Cheyne-Stokes respiration. That usually means that there is some sort of metabolic problem. Diabetes. Liver failure. Kidney failure. Not a hemorrhage."

"We'll see. I ordered everything."

Just then the phone rang. It was the lab technician. He had some results. He read them out to Dr. MacMillan.

Sugar: 110. Bonnie wasn't in a diabetic coma.

BUN: 10. That ruled out kidney failure.

Creatinine: 0.9. So did that.

The list of what she didn't have was growing.

Liver enzymes: normal. That made acute liver failure highly unlikely.

Calcium: normal. She had not had a seizure because her calcium level was too low.

Her magnesium level was normal.

Sodium: 100.

"What?" MacMillan yelled.

"One hundred," the technician replied.

"Give me the rest of the electrolytes."

The technician did.

They were all very low. Far below normal.

"What's in that IV?" he yelled as he hung up the phone.

"Five percent glucose."

"How many bottles has she had?"

"This is number eight."

"All just sugar water?"

"All just sugar water. That's what Greengrass ordered."

"He ordered all those?"

"Five percent glucose. One liter every two hours," she said, quoting the admission order verbatim.

"Eight bottles. No wonder her sodium hit a hundred. God! I hope we can save her."

So did Grace. She'd put up several of those bottles and never questioned the order.

"Damn it. Get some saline."

"Half normal?"

"No. The strongest you have."

"All I have is normal."

"Hang it. And get some ten percent up here. Now. STAT."

Grace ran to carry out his orders. She, too, now understood exactly what had happened. And why. If only it wasn't too late. Bonnie had been admitted because of hyperemesis gravidarum. She had been vomiting and losing weight and was dehydrated. That meant she had lost fluid. She needed fluid. But not just water. She had lost both water and salts. And all they had given her was water with some sugar in it. Too much water. And as they flooded her with water, the relative amount of sodium in her body went down. Too far. Grace had never seen a patient with a sodium below 110. No, she had once, during training — 108. That patient had died.

Bonnie Lawrence did not die.

Within six hours, MacMillan had gotten her sodium level back to normal. And all her other levels, too. And she did not die. But she didn't recover, either. In a few days the family was told that she would never get any better. She had gone into a coma because of her hyperemesis gravidarum. That was why Dr. Greengrass had told her to call if she lost four more pounds. He had been very worried. She hadn't called until it was too late.

They knew all that. They wanted an expert opinion on what to expect in the future. They wanted an expert on the brain to see her, a neurologist, just to make certain that everything possible was being done for her, and someone who could tell them about her future course.

That was how I got called in. At first, I didn't want to see her at all. I doubted that there was a damn thing I could do to help her.

But her husband persuaded me to see her. She was so young. Just
a few days before she had been normal, and now her doctors were
all but calling her a vegetable.

I went to see her.

She was not as advertised. She was not in a coma. Nor was she
a "vegetable." That term is sometimes used to describe patients
who are in a chronic vegetative state — a state in which the patient,
because of severe brain damage, can only perform vegetative functions. The lungs breathe. The heart beats. The blood pressure is
maintained. The kidneys work. The liver does, too. So does the
gastrointestinal system, but not the brain. Like a vegetable.

Mrs. Lawrence was not a vegetable. She was not in coma.

I knew that the moment I walked into the room. Her eyes were
open. No one in coma keeps the eyes open.

I called to her.

She made no response. No movement at all.

I called her again.

No movement. No response. She didn't open her mouth as if to
speak. She didn't move her eyes. Nothing moved.

I tried a different stimulus. Pain. I rubbed my knuckles up and
down her sternum.

Nothing happened. It was as if she didn't feel a thing. Like a
vegetable.

I took out my flashlight and shined it in her right eye. The pupil
constricted promptly. I got the same response on the left. So what?
That was a simple, primitive reflex. No big deal. A vegetable with
a simple reflex.

I moved the light to the left.

Her eyes did not move.

I moved the light the other way.

Once again her eyes continued to stare straight ahead.

I had only one more trick to try before I pronounced her a
vegetable. I moved the light upward.

And her eyes followed it.

They moved.

Upward.

Then I moved my light down.

Below the vertical plane.

And once again her eyes followed the light.

Down.

Up and down they went, following my flashlight.

But not side to side.

She was not in coma.

She was not a vegetable.

She was locked in. Her brain could still direct her eyes to move up and down, but it could not direct any other movement.

Why not?

Of all the movements of the body — all of which are directed by the brain — vertical eye movements are located nearest to the brain itself, in the upper part of the brain stem. If all that the patient can do is move the eyes up and down, then the brain is cut off from the rest of the nervous system just below the center for vertical eye movements. Movement cannot take place below that. And sensation below that cannot get up to the brain. The rest is cut off, locked away, and the brain is locked in.

Light stimulus gets into the brain above the level of the cut. It enters the eyes and goes to the brain and the brain, like that of a simple primitive animal, follows that light.

Up and down.

Not a vegetable.

But was enough of her brain left functioning that good use could be made of her one remaining function?

Could she respond to simple verbal commands?

Did sounds get up to her brain?

And if so, could she put together a meaningful response? Could she move her eyes on command? If she could, then she could communicate her needs, her feelings.

If not, she would not be much better off than a vegetable. And maybe worse off. Capable of some understanding. Some feeling, some emotion. And not able to respond.

Locked in.

"Move your eyes up," I said.

No response.

"Move your eyes up," I begged.

"Move your eyes up," I implored.

"Move your eyes up," I prayed.

I tried the same with down.

Nothing happened.

I saw her every other day for two weeks. She never changed. She remained locked in. Totally locked in.

My consult was short and straightforward: Bonnie had a locked-in syndrome due to destruction of the pons. That's the area just below the centers for vertical gaze.

The lesion in her pons was what is called "central pontine myelinolysis." All that means is that there is a big hole in the pons preventing all messages from getting in or out and thus locking her in.

Her CPM had been the result of her severely low sodium level.

Her low sodium level had been caused by water intoxication. She had received excessive water without sodium, as a result of the orders of Dr. Greengrass.

And she would never get any better.

All in one sentence.

Permanent locked-in syndrome secondary to CPM due to iatrogenic water intoxication.

I stopped seeing her and never gave her another thought until two years later. I got a call from a lawyer. His name was Harry Walker. He represented the Lawrences in a malpractice suit against Dr. Greengrass and the hospital. Would I be willing to act as an expert witness?

I hesitated.

Did I know the role of an expert witness?

Yes.

How? Had I appeared in any malpractice cases?

No. Just in one personal injury case.

The role of an expert was the same in both, but the nature of what had to be proved was a bit different. In malpractice, which was really a form of professional negligence, two things had to be proved. The first was professional negligence.

"Meaning?"

"A deviation from the standard of care."

"Meaning?"

"Doing something that was not an acceptable part of medical care."

"You mean like giving a patient so much water intravenously that you can cause water intoxication?"

"Yes. You recall the case."

"Very well."

He then went on to explain that any such deviation could be either a sin of commission — writing the order for one liter of water every two hours forever — or a sin of omission, the failure to do something.

"Like the nurses not calling him after two or three bottles to get a change of orders."

"Yes."

Would I be willing to be an expert on standard of care?

"Yes."

The second element, of course, was causation. Had the deviation led to damage?

In Bonnie's case, the answer was obvious.

"Permanent locked-in syndrome secondary to CPM due to iatrogenic water intoxication," I said.

"Would I say that in court?"

"Yes."

"As an expert?"

"Yes."

"They will put pressure on you."

"Who?"

"Other doctors, the Dean's office."

"Why?"

"Doctors don't like doctors to testify against other doctors."

"I'm not testifying against another doctor," I said innocently. "I'm testifying for Bonnie Lawrence. She was a normal, healthy woman who was turned into a vegetable by a doctor's mistake."

"Deviation from the standard of care."

"That's what I meant. She deserves her day in court. And to have that day in court, she has to have an expert witness."

"That's right, Doc."

"It's the only way she can get justice. And it's probably the only way those of us who believe in maintaining an appropriate standard of practice can express ourselves."

"But they will put pressure on you."

"I doubt it."

The case moved forward rather quickly. The defense took my deposition. It focused on both elements of the case, since I was acting as an expert on both negligence and causation.

Causation was rather obvious. No one could deny that before her sodium bottomed out at about one hundred, Bonnie's brain had been normal, and now she was "locked in." I testified as to causation. So did MacMillan, who had treated her after having been called in by Greengrass.

Bonnie had had an abnormally low sodium level.

How low?

As low as either of us had ever seen.

What had caused the low sodium?

"Water intoxication," I said. "From all the salt-free water Greengrass had given her."

MacMillan commented about sodium loss from vomiting, but when pressed, had said the same thing I did. "Water intoxication."

The "water intoxication," I testified, caused her locked-in syndrome. And her status was permanent.

Next came the questions of deviation from the standard of care.

Had anyone been guilty of a deviation from the standard of care?

Yes.

Who?

I started with Greengrass.

Was I an obstetrician?

No.

Then how could I pretend to know the standard of care provided by obstetricians?

I wasn't commenting on his obstetrical activities, but on his care of a dehydrated patient. And he had to meet the standard of care of any physician for this problem and hadn't.

His deviations were obvious. He had given Bonnie water without sodium, at an enormous rate, had never changed his order, and had never gone to see her.

Was anyone else guilty?

The nurses.

Why?

They continued to follow his orders and did not make sure that he or some other doctor actually saw the patient.

Anyone else?

No.

MacMillan?

No.

End of deposition.

Two days later, as I was walking to the parking lot, the executive vice president of the hospital stopped me. He was also a surgeon.

"Do you know Harry Walker?" he asked me.

"Yes."

"He's a bad guy," he said.

"Why?"

"He makes life hard for all of us."

"Oh."

"Malpractice rates are much too high."

"I see. But sometimes doctors do screw up."

He shrugged his shoulders.

"What should such patients do?"

"No one cares if you appear in a case every few years," he said, "but stay away from Walker and his kind."

I nodded.

"And make sure you only testify in cases involving little hospitals, like this Lawrence case. We don't like to be involved with anything that involves the big hospitals in Chicago."

"I see," I said. "I can be on the side of truth and justice as long as I testify for the defense or only against little hospitals."

"That's not what I said."

"Isn't it?"

"And I never even saw you today." With that, he walked away.

That was 1975. The case never came to trial. The Lawrences got about one and a half million, half from Greengrass (or really his insurance company) and half from the hospital via its insurance company. The medical community thought that the Lawrences had won and organized medicine had somehow lost. I was considered a turncoat. A piranha. To them, it had not been a game.

And everyone had lost. The Lawrences certainly had not won. No matter how much money they might have gotten, they had lost. And lost big.

But I felt good about what I had done. I didn't delude myself. The level of care would not suddenly get better. Doctors would not all of a sudden be more careful in treating women with hyperemesis gravidarum, but Greengrass probably would, and the nurses at his hospital certainly would.

And the Lawrences had "gotten their day in court." Without an expert, that couldn't have happened.

Bonnie was still locked in.

Still little more than a vegetable.

But now she could get the best care that money could buy.

The day the case was settled, Harry Walker called me to thank me and ask me a question. Would I be willing to look at another case?

Why not?

He reminded me of my conversation with the executive vice president.

How had the vice president known about my acting as an expert?

The same people insure many hospitals, and all their defense firms work together. And my appearance in a deposition is part of the public record. If I ever appeared again, everyone would know.

"Send me the record," I said. "I don't respond well to threats."

AUTHOR'S NOTE

As I was compiling these reminiscences, I was struck by my degree of naïveté. I was innocent enough to believe that by testifying for what I knew to be true in a malpractice case, I could do some real good. I was wrong. Acting as an expert witness for plaintiffs does not help the medical establishment eliminate or control incompetent physicians. After all, most malpractice does not involve the worst of medical practitioners, but average doctors who have made a mistake. And even those few physicians who are sued over and over again rarely, if ever, lose staff privileges at a hospital. If their ability to practice medicine is ever curbed, it is only by the insurance companies who finally cut off their insurance.

CHAPTER THREE

Waving Good-bye

Today, I am the happiest man alive.

> — Lou Gehrig, *in a farewell speech to fans gathered in Yankee Stadium for Lou Gehrig Day, following his retirement from baseball because of amyotrophic lateral sclerosis.*

Tom Thompson III had never worked this hard in his entire life, nor been as happy. His years of hard work were at last paying off. He was not rich. He might never be rich, but he no longer had to worry about the future. And it had only taken him four years, not the eight to ten years he had figured it would take. Four years earlier, his father had finally retired, and Tom had taken over the family business. And none too soon.

The family business was a laundry service, the oldest one in Memphis. It had been started, around the turn of the century, by Tom Thompson's grandfather, the first Tommy Thompson, who did laundry for hotels and restaurants. Then his dad had taken over, adding hospitals to their clientele. For decades things went along smoothly. But times changed. Hotels changed hands. So did hospitals. Cost containment became the ruling principle. Hotels and hospitals started doing their own laundry. The competition became more aggressive with faster service. Dad couldn't keep up. Business declined. Bankruptcy seemed just around the corner.

In four years he had turned that all around. Modernization, aggressive marketing, and new, shiny delivery trucks led to new customers, faster service, competitive contracts. Two large hospitals closed their own laundries and signed long-term contracts. Tom Thompson had opened a second laundry facility, and a third was on the drawing boards.

Success.

Financial security.

But at a cost. He was exhausted both emotionally and physically. He worked sixteen hours a day, six days a week. And he hadn't had a vacation in those four years. His emotional exhaustion was apparent to everyone: his wife, their two kids, his friends, his secretary. He was more curt and short-tempered than he had ever been, with everyone. His physical exhaustion was apparent only to him. He still ran three miles every day, but it took him longer: thirty-five minutes, not twenty-four. And his left leg seemed to drag, especially during that third mile.

And his muscles twitched. He could feel the twitches, or ripples, as he called them. First in one arm, then the other, then in a leg. Especially the left leg. The muscle rippled. He could feel the twitches and, if he looked, see them, like the rippling of the muscles of a horse just before a race. Except his were worse after he ran.

He deserved a vacation. He needed a vacation. Two weeks away from work. Two weeks sun with nothing to do but sit in sun and relax and play a little tennis and make love to his wife.

They went to the Club Med in the Bahamas. It was wonderful. The kids had their own activities, and the adults were free to do what they wanted. And Tom and Jill did just that. Tom had never felt more relaxed. He had never been happier. They had never made love more often. It was just what they both needed, precisely what he needed. Just what the doctor ordered. He felt great except for his left leg. It seemed to drag more and more. It was so bad that Jill was beating him in tennis, every set. He couldn't even hold his own serve.

Once he got home, he went to see his doctor. Dr. Burke had been their family doctor for years. He listened to Tom's story and told him that he had better see a neurologist.

Any particular neurologist?

His doctor recommended Manfred Schmidt. Tom saw him the next day. And told him his story. Dr. Schmidt was interested in two aspects. The left leg and the "ripples."

Schmidt asked him about dozens of possible symptoms. Numbness? Tingling? Trouble seeing? Trouble with his bladder? Many more. Tom had none of them. At first, that made him feel good.

All he had were ripples and a foot that dragged. Everything else in his nervous system seemed to be working fine. But as the list got longer, Tom became increasingly uncomfortable. Were these symptoms he was expected to have or that were going to develop? And if so, when? How soon?

Then Tom went into an examining room, undressed, and put on an ill-fitting gown that seemed to have been designed to fit no one and that required an advanced degree in structural engineering to close. Dr. Schmidt examined him as he had never been examined before. With a flashlight. A rubber hammer. A tuning fork. A safety pin. A cotton wisp. God knows what else.

In the end, he told Tom that Tom's left foot dragged and that he had ripples.

Tom already knew that much.

Although Schmidt used a different word. He called the ripples "fasciculations."

"But what do I have?" Tom asked.

"I don't know. We must do some simple tests."

Tom was all for that. The nurse drew some blood and gave him a bottle so he could collect his urine for twenty-four hours, and Tom was given an appointment for an EMG to be done by Dr. Schmidt the next afternoon.

The EMG was not a "simple" test. At least not for the patient. Dr. Schmidt spent the better part of an hour sticking thin needles into Tom's muscles. And not just in the left foot. Both feet. Both legs. Both arms. Both hands. His back. And then sending jolts of electricity up and down his nerves. Both arms. Both hands. Both legs.

When the test was over, Dr. Schmidt smiled at him and said, "Come back next week so we can go over all your tests."

Tom nodded.

"And bring your wife."

Tom did not have to ask him why.

The next week passed by as if it were no more than a decade or two. Each day he went to work and worked a mere ten to twelve hours. Each night he went home and didn't run. He ate dinner. He watched TV. And he went to bed and didn't make love to Jill. He was too busy counting fasciculations and remembering the list of symptoms that he was now certain he would some day develop:

Trouble talking.

Swallowing difficulty.

Incontinence.

Impotence.

Breathing problems.

Jill went with Tom to see Dr. Schmidt. It was Jill who asked the doctor if he knew what was wrong with Tom.

He did.

What exactly?

"Amyotrophic lateral sclerosis. A.L.S."

Neither Tom nor Jill knew exactly what that was.

"Lou Gehrig's disease," the doctor explained.

They knew what that was.

And Dr. Schmidt told them exactly what that meant. Progressive weakness. Inexorably progressive. Spreading throughout Tom's body. Legs. Arms. Face. Swallowing. Speech. Breathing.

By then, neither of them really heard what he was saying.

Pneumonia.

Aspiration.

"How long?" Jill finally asked.

It was difficult to be certain.

"How long?" she asked again.

"Two years — three at the most."

"Oh God," she gasped.

"Are you sure?" Tom asked.

He was.

"How . . . ?"

"The fasciculations," Dr. Schmidt replied.

"My ripples."

"Yes. Those ripples, as you call them, are caused by abnormal discharges of your motor nerve cells in the spinal cord. Those cells are the cells that die in A.L.S., and as they die, they cause these fasciculations. Those ripples show us that the cells are dying."

Jill was crying softly.

Tom felt a ripple in his right arm. The motor cells in his spinal cord were deteriorating. This was their way of waving good-bye.

Was there any treatment?

No. None.

Was there anything he could do?

Exercise. Stay in as good shape as possible.

Anything else?

Dr. Schmidt just shrugged his shoulders.

Weren't there other tests to do?

No.

Was he certain?

He was.

Why?

The fasciculations.

His cells waving good-bye.

That night Jill wanted to make love.

Tom didn't.

She persisted.

He became aroused. At least he could still get aroused. And get an erection. And make love to his wife. It felt so good. He was still alive. He could still function as a man. As a husband. As a lover.

He felt a ripple in his right arm.

At least his penis wasn't waving good-bye. Not yet.

But it was.

He lost his erection.

Jill tried to fight back her tears but couldn't. They held each other and cried together.

The next morning, Jill called Dr. Schmidt and explained what had happened.

"Depression," he said. It was to be expected.

What should she do?

Be supportive. Remain interested but not make too many demands.

She thought she understood.

Tom went in to work that day. But it wasn't just another day at work. He spent the day in meetings. Not with his foreman, or sales personnel, or drivers, but with his lawyer, accountant, and broker (who called himself a financial advisor).

By five o'clock, Tom had a plan for the rest of his life. All two or three years of it. He and Jill talked about it after they had put the kids to bed. He would sell the business. It was making money. There were buyers who were interested. If he had five more years, he was certain they could get four times as much. The new plants would both be operational. By then, the new hotels would be open, the cash flow would be far greater, and the profit.

But he didn't have five years.

And there was no one else to run the business. He had to think of Jill and the two kids.

So he would sell the business, and stay on as a consultant — with a salary and health insurance. And they would put the money in an annuity. She and the kids would be provided for. Not extravagantly, but they would get by. And he would have more time to spend with them as a father.

Good time, time beginning now, not at the end when he could hardly move. But now.

It seemed like a good plan to Jill.

That night they went to sleep holding hands. Tom didn't try to make love to Jill. And she didn't try to make love to him.

It, of course, took several months to arrange everything. It all worked out much as Tom had imagined it. Once the papers were signed, it was as if a great burden had been taken from his shoulders.

His leg was weaker. It dragged all the time. But he was no longer anxious. No longer worried whenever he looked at Jill or the kids. He was no longer so depressed. He ate with more appetite, played with the kids for hours on end, and after dinner he and Jill would rehash each and every event of the day.

It was not like old times. It was far better. Old times had never been like this. Tom had always worked so hard. Now he had more time for her and the children and more energy. And more enthusiasm.

It was time to try again.

She started it.

He responded. He responded fully. He entered her and then dissolved.

Neither of them talked about it. Perhaps he was still depressed. Still preoccupied. Who could blame him? Not Jill. He was doing so well. Still, she wanted so much to make love with him, to share that intimacy, to bring him that joy.

Two weeks later she tried again. More slowly. More tenderly. She even took him in her mouth for a while. Tom had always liked that. But it didn't help. The same result. Tom felt ashamed. Defeated. Angry. Jill was certain she had hurt him deeply.

She called Dr. Schmidt and told him the problem. Was it the . . . A.L.S.?

"No."

Did he want to examine Tom again?

"In a month."

And in the meantime?

"See a psychiatrist. He's depressed."

It took two weeks for Jill to broach the subject of seeing a psychiatrist. Tom didn't seem depressed to her. In fact, he seemed to be doing remarkably well. He and their son were building a race car together. He had built a doll house for their daughter. Next would be a bird feeder to go outside the kitchen window.

Maybe it was her problem.

Maybe she didn't excite him anymore.

Finally one night as they lay in bed, she asked him.

No. It wasn't that. He loved her. Her body still excited him. He just couldn't. It was his disease.

She told him that Dr. Schmidt told her that it wasn't the A.L.S. That surprised him.

She told him what Dr. Schmidt had suggested.

Three days later Tom saw the psychiatrist, a Dr. Bednarik. In the next week, he had three visits with him, then the three of them met for a conference. The psychiatrist hadn't seen many patients with A.L.S. In fact, Tom was the first. But he'd seen lots of patients with depression. Hundreds of them. And in his opinion, Tom was not depressed. He thought that Tom was doing remarkably well from a psychiatric viewpoint. Few patients ever came to terms with their own mortality quite so well as Tom had. The doctor wanted Tom to work with groups of patients who had similar problems. Patients with other terminal illnesses.

"His impotence?" Jill asked.

Talk to Dr. Schmidt.

They did just that — one week later. Schmidt took a history again. He asked his same questions.

Numbness?

Swallowing difficulties?

Breathing?

Impotence?

That one got a positive response.

Weakness?

So did that.

Where?

Both legs.

Jill was shocked. She hadn't realized that both legs were now weak. That his disease was progressing. No wonder Tom didn't feel up to being a lover.

Schmidt examined Tom. He confirmed what they both knew — weakness of both feet.

Schmidt said nothing more.

Tom asked him about his impotence.

"We see that sometimes."

"Isn't there anything else to do? More tests? Any medications? Anything?"

Schmidt merely shook his head.

"When should I come back?"

"Every three months."

It was June. The kids were out of school. Tom knew just what he wanted to do for the summer. Each day his legs were getting weaker. At the rate the weakness was progressing, he figured he'd be in a wheelchair by the fall. Tom had family and friends spread over the country, from Maine to California. People who were important to him. People he wanted to see once more while he was still fairly healthy. He did not want them to see him later when his entire body was deteriorating, when people would no longer see him as Tom Thompson, but as the victim of a tragic fate.

They borrowed a recreational van from some good friends and had the pedals fixed so that it could be driven by someone who could not use his legs, and off they went. Tom's college roommate, Paul Van Buren, lived in Maine. They started there. Paul was married to his college sweetheart. They also had two children. Jill had called ahead to let them know what had happened to Tom, what was happening to him every day, and what would happen to him in the future. Neither she nor Tom wanted any sympathy, but she didn't want there to be any uncomfortable surprises.

And there weren't. It went better than either Tom or Jill had expected. Paul was just what Tom needed. Supportive, but not fawning. They reminisced without getting maudlin.

They had planned on staying in Maine for three days and ended up staying two weeks. They might have stayed longer, but that last night Tom felt better than he had in months. True, his legs were weaker. They both dragged now and he could hardly lift them into the van without using his hands. But he was less anxious about the future. Jill and the kids were provided for. And they had good friends who could help them through the tough times. And Jill was always there, doing the right thing, saying the right thing.

He loved her so.

He wanted so to make love to her.

For the first time since Schmidt had pronounced those three letters, he really felt like making love to his wife.

He rolled over in bed and began kissing her and fondling her. And nothing happened.

Nothing at all.

Not even an inkling of a response.

A.L.S. was not just three letters. It was a progressive torture.

Tom needed a change of scenery.

Off to Philadelphia and a slew of cousins and several assorted uncles and aunts.

Jill, of course, had once again forewarned everyone, but his aunts were too solicitous and his cousins seemed to oscillate between worries that A.L.S. might turn out to be contagious or hereditary and a state of pity. Philadelphia lasted only three days.

Jill had relatives in Pittsburgh — two days. While there, she called Schmidt and told him about the total impotence.

"Don't you people ever think of anything other than sex?" he retorted.

She felt ashamed to have bothered him.

Tom had some friends, business acquaintances really, in Chicago. And an uncle. And he had always wanted to see the sights. As a family, they went to the Art Institute, the Museum of Science and Industry, the Field Museum, the aquarium, the planetarium, and the beaches. In the museum, Tom sat whenever he could, while Jill took the children from room to room, from exhibit to exhibit. He learned that if you sat in the middle of each room in the Art Institute and waited long enough, you could eventually see every picture that was hanging in that room as the crowds came and went. Even *American Gothic* and *Sunday Afternoon on the Grand Jatte*, although he never saw all of the latter at once. There was always at least one person between him and Seurat. Neither Tom nor Jill ever talked about his impotence nor his weakness, which was getting worse every day.

They bought a cane. It didn't help.

On Friday night, they went out to dinner with Don Paul, the senior partner of the firm that had bought him out. Don lived in Chicago. He was fifty, a stickler for details, and a fastidious dresser. Tom had not grown fond of him during their negotiations. The Pauls were not his choice for dinner partners, but Don had left a message in Atlanta that he wanted to talk to Tom, and the office manager had tracked him down. He had no choice.

The four of them went out to dinner. They met at one of the city's fanciest French restaurants. Jill had bought a dress for the occasion. At Marshall Fields. Tom had bought a new shirt and a tie. He hadn't brought a tie with him. When they got to the Ciel Bleu, the Pauls were waiting for them. Tom could see that Don was shocked by Tom's disability. Tom, too, was shocked by it. There were three stairs in the restaurant. Without Jill's help, he could never have climbed them. The cane didn't help. He would soon need a wheelchair. Or a walker. Or a pair of sherpas. And then what?

After they sat down, the atmosphere began to improve. Tom was no longer a freak or a cripple. It was almost as if he were normal. He could use his hands and arms just like a normal person. He could eat. He could feed himself. He could swallow without dribbling. Or choking.

For how long, he wondered.

Don talked about business.

Tom hardly listened. He thought about swallowing difficulties. And pneumonia. Jill smiled and nodded politely. Tom wondered if she was even listening to Don.

Mrs. Paul was the second Mrs. Paul. Her first name was Connie. She was a twenty-four-year-old, tall, thin blonde who hung on her husband's words and kept fingering her diamond ring. She had a stunning figure, especially for someone that thin.

Tom was certain that Don wasn't impotent.

It was over dessert that Don made Tom an offer. They were buying another family laundry business in Birmingham, but it was nowhere near as well run or as well organized as Tom's had been. Would he be willing to help them reorganize it?

Tom wasn't sure. He wanted to spend his time with his family.

Don offered him an equity position in the venture. That made it tempting. It was their time together versus greater financial security.

Tom was interested.

Don was pleased. They would go out on his boat Sunday afternoon and work out the details. Don ordered a bottle of champagne to celebrate. Dom Perignon. What else?

It was as he got up to leave that the trouble became evident. Tom got up from his chair all by himself — a minor triumph, but as he did, he realized that his pants were wet.

He had not spilled any champagne.

Or water.

He had wet himself.

Like a baby.

Or a demented old fool.

Incontinence.

Had anyone else noticed?

Jill was talking to Don. Neither of them was looking at him. Connie was.

He looked at her and stared into her large blue eyes. She fluttered her eyelids. She looked like a Barbie Doll, a vacuous Barbie Doll without a real thought in her head.

She stared back very briefly, then took out a compact and lifted it in front of her face. Without breaking her concentration, she began to talk.

"I know a very good neurologist. His name is Klawans. I don't know if he can help you or not. He helped my sister." She went on to give him my office address and tell him how to get my phone number.

Tom had already seen one neurologist too many.

Saturday morning Tom went out and bought a wheelchair. While he was out, Jill called Dr. Schmidt.

"Are you calling about that sex business again?"

"No. His legs are weaker."

"That is what is to be expected."

"And he wet his pants at dinner."

"You must learn to live with such things. He's going to get worse." Schmidt began to describe the progression of the disease. Jill hung up and made another phone call. She called the Pauls. Connie answered. Don was out. Jill said that they wouldn't be coming on Sunday.

Connie understood. She told Jill what she'd observed. "Don didn't notice," Connie said. "And I didn't tell him. When he's talking about business, he never notices me unless I take off all my clothes."

"Thanks for not telling him, but I doubt if Tom wants to take the chance again."

"He might be able to use a Texas catheter."

"A what?"

Connie explained. She had a sister with M.S. She had to have a regular catheter in her bladder, but men could use a Texas catheter. It was like a condom. It fit right over. "I gave your husband the name of a neurologist."

"Who?"

She told Jill my name.

That Thursday, I got a phone call from Duluth. It was after five; my secretary had gone home for the day. She usually protects me from calls from people who aren't patients of mine, but who somehow get my name and call up for information, but she wasn't there, so I answered the phone.

It was a Mrs. Thompson. Her husband had Lou Gehrig's disease.

I knew I was not going to enjoy the conversation. I dislike both the disease and the eponym; the disease because there is virtually nothing I can do for its victim except make the correct diagnosis and then watch the motor nerve cells wave good-bye, the eponym because it's too parochial. Lou Gehrig died from A.L.S. And I guess using his name in this country may help raise money, but neurology is international. No one outside the U.S. has any idea who Lou Gehrig was or what disease destroyed his career and then his life. It would be just as appropriate if the French called syphilis of the nervous system Guy de Maupassant's disease, while the Germans called it Heinrich Heine's disease.

"A.L.S.," I replied.

"Yes. Can I ask you a few questions?"

Either my secretary had to work later, or I had to stop answering the phone. "Of course."

"What is A.L.S.?"

I sat down, took a deep breath, and began my first-year lecture on degenerative diseases of the central nervous system. A.L.S. is a progressive disease of the brain and spinal cord. The cause is totally unknown. There is no known treatment. It is a fatal disease. The cells continue to die off until . . .

That much she knew. Too well. She hesitated.

"Then why did you call?"

"Which cells?"

"The motor cells," I began, and then explained that there are two types of such cells, the upper motor neurons and the lower motor neurons. The upper motor neurons are in the brain. They carry messages from the brain to the lower motor neurons. They initiate and control movement. As they become diseased, the patient has difficulty initiating and performing movements — progressive paralysis with stiffness, which we call spasticity, and increased reflexes. The lower motor neurons are in the brain stem. They receive instructions from the upper motor neurons and, in turn, direct the muscles to perform movements. As they die, the muscles become weak and lose bulk, a process we'll call atrophy, and as they are dying, the muscles have spontaneous ripples.

"Fasciculations," she said.

"Yes."

"Is that all?"

I wasn't sure what she meant. After all, I had described a fatal process. As the lower motor nerves in the spinal cord die out, the patient loses the ability to walk. An inexorable process — cane — wheelchair — bed. Progressive loss of function of the arms. Progressive inability to breathe. And as the lower motor cells in the brain stem fail, things get even worse — inability to talk, to chew, to swallow.

Aspiration.

Choking.

Pneumonia.

She knew all that, she again informed me. "What else?"

"Nothing."

"Incontinence?"

"No. Not unless the patient can't get to the bathroom."

"Impotence?"

"No."

"Are you sure?"

"Yes."

"Thank you," she said, about to hang up.

I stopped her and asked her again why she had called me. She told me about her husband.

"He may not have A.L.S.," I said.

"But his doctor . . ."

"Doctors can be wrong. Is he there with you?"

He was.

"Ask him how he knew he'd wet his pants. Did he see it? Or feel it?"

I could hear their muffled conversation.

"He saw it."

"Is he sure of that?"

More muffled words.

"Yes."

"He doesn't have A.L.S. That kind of sensory loss where he can't feel himself urinating and can't feel the wet urine is not part of A.L.S."

"What does he have?"

"I can't be sure."

"Can he be cured?"

Without knowing what he had, I couldn't answer that.

"What could it be?"

It was probably a spinal cord tumor, but listing all the possible diagnoses of what a patient might have is never very helpful to patients. So I told her I didn't know but that he needed to be reevaluated immediately.

She thanked me and hung up.

That, I assumed, would be my first and last contact with her. I was wrong. Four weeks later, they appeared in my office. After Mrs. Thompson had ended our conversation, she'd called Dr. Schmidt and told him what she had learned.

He was infuriated. How could she listen to some doctor who'd never even examined her husband? He had examined him. He had done an EMG. If they wanted, he would do another. It wouldn't help. Lou Gehrig's disease was fatal. "One hundred percent of the time."

"But impotence."

"He's depressed. I would be, too, if I had that disease."

"And incontinence."

"How often?"

"Once."

"Hm. Tell me about it."

She did.

"It's no big deal. Too much to drink."

"But he didn't feel . . ."

"Too much alcohol."

"What should I do? Should we see another neurologist?"

"It's your money, but I wouldn't waste it on some jerk who makes diagnoses over the phone."

Two days later, Tom again lost his urine and wet his pants. And he hadn't been drinking at all. And then once more the next day.

Once again she called Dr. Schmidt.

"So what," he replied. "It's nothing new. He was incontinent before, wasn't he?"

"Yes."

"Nothing ever gets better in this disease."

Tom began to dribble urine. Jill bought some Texas catheters. When she put the first one on, Tom tried to make a joke. "And you thought I'd never be able to use a condom again."

Jill didn't laugh, but she walked out of the room before she allowed herself to cry.

He had been using a Texas catheter for almost two weeks when I saw him. An episode of soiling his pants had resulted in the decision to seek another opinion.

Better late than never, I said to myself.

The history was clear-cut: progressive weakness of the legs for less than a year. He now used a wheelchair all the time.

Was there any arm weakness?

No.

None at all?

No.

Swallowing difficulty — no.

Speech — none.

Choking — none.

After the weakness, he developed impotence, progressing from partial to total.

And then incontinence. First urinary. Then fecal.

"And sensory loss," I added.

"Yes. I can't really feel my belt."

"From the waist down?"

"No. I can feel my knees."

The exam confirmed the history.

"You don't have A.L.S.," I told him.

"But the fasciculations?" they both protested.

"What fasciculations?" (I didn't see any.)

"I haven't had them in months," he realized.

"Did you feel them?"

"Yes."

"Did they go away when you stopped working so hard?"

"Yes."

"Those weren't true fasciculations. They were pseudofasciculations. Lots of people have them. They come out with fatigue and overwork."

"What does my husband have?" Jill interrupted.

"I think he has a tumor at the base of the spinal cord."

"Why?" she asked.

"Everything above the waist is normal. And everything below is abnormal. Motor. Sensory. Reflexes. Bladder control. Sexual function. There is something there involving all the systems. That's what tumors do."

"Can you help him?"

"I hope so."

I admitted him to our hospital that day. The next day we did a CT scan of the spine and a myelogram and saw the tumor, and that afternoon, a neurosurgeon removed it.

It was a benign tumor. No cancer. No malignancy. Once the neurosurgeon removed the bone and got down to the tumor, it almost fell out by itself.

Tom was cured.

But he didn't get much better. His incontinence never improved. Nor his impotence. Nor his weakness. He could feel his belt and his thighs — not a major triumph. He left the hospital in a wheelchair, wearing a Texas catheter.

The last time I saw him in the hospital, he asked me a couple of questions.

If the diagnosis had been made earlier, would he be better off?

Of course. Removing the tumor cured him. And the removal was easy. The tumor all but jumped out. It was benign. If he'd been operated on while he could still walk, he'd still be walking.

"And before I was incontinent?"

"No incontinence."

"And before I was impotent?"

"No impotence."

"Then I'd have a real use for a condom."

I nodded.

"Should Dr. Schmidt have made the diagnosis?"

"He should have looked," I replied.

Many fellow physicians criticize me for this and similar responses. Not that it wasn't the most honest answer that I could give, but that I was causing a problem for Dr. Schmidt and all of organized medicine. Or at least "neurology."

Perhaps I was. So be it.

Thompson and Thompson v. Schmidt was the title of the case. It never came to trial. I did give a deposition, however, as an expert for the plaintiffs. My testimony covered two aspects of the matter. Deviation from the standard of care — negligence on the part of Dr. Schmidt — and the damage caused by his deviation from the standard of care.

My testimony, I thought, was precise. It was given in my office. Since I was an expert for the plaintiffs, the lawyer for the defense asked the questions. He was in his late forties, well dressed, smooth in both appearance and demeanor. Juries would not like him, but they would trust him. He brought Dr. Schmidt with him. Schmidt was in his late fifties; he wore a five-hundred-dollar suit, and a large diamond on his little finger. There was a permanent sneer on his face. He stared at me continuously, which was supposed to make me uncomfortable. It didn't. I pretended he was a first-year resident who needed to learn some neurology. I hoped he was educable. I doubted it. Juries, I concluded, would not like him.

His lawyer was named Angsman.

He started by asking my opinions and letting me outline what I believed, as if he really wanted to hear what I had to say, what I would say if I got in front of a jury.

"Dr. Schmidt should have evaluated Mr. Thompson for a tumor of the spinal cord the first time he saw him."

"How?"

"By performing a myelogram."

"Would that have demonstrated the tumor?"

"Yes."

"And the surgery should have been done then, at that time?"

"Yes."

"And that would have avoided all future injury?"

"Yes."

"And left Mr. Thompson with only a drag of his left leg?"

"Yes."

"No incontinence?"

"No."

"No impotence?"

"None."

"Was it also a deviation not to do the myelogram once Mr. Thompson developed the first symptom of partial impotence?"

"Absolutely."

"And if it had been done then, would it have shown the tumor?"

"Most definitely."

"And surgery would have prevented any progression?"

"Certainly."

"No wheelchair?"

"None."

"No incontinence?"

"Absolutely not."

"And his impotence?"

"Most likely would have disappeared."

"Normal sexual function?"

"More probably than not."

So it went. With each added symptom, Dr. Schmidt should have realized that the patient needed a myelogram, deserved a myelogram. Each time he failed to do one, his negligence continued. Of course, his maintaining that the added symptoms were due to A.L.S. was bad neurology and not true. That assumption was what kept him from doing the myelogram. It was part and parcel of the same negligence.

So much for my opinions. Short but not very sweet. Dr. Schmidt was still staring at me. His sneer was gone. It had been replaced by a glare of utter hatred. I smiled back at him. He turned and whispered into Angsman's ear. They whispered back and forth for a couple of minutes. It was then that Angsman went to work on me.

Had I read the depositions of the defense experts?

I had.

"Dr. Harder?"

"Yes."

"Do you agree that he is a distinguished expert on spinal-cord tumor?"

"Yes."

"Do you disagree with his opinions?"

"No." I had read his deposition. He was an honest man who had given honest answers to the wrong questions. I was sure his opinion was the same as mine. He just hadn't been asked the right question. Not yet, at least. And the difference was not just in semantics. It was not a game of words. It was the truth about how medicine should be practiced.

"Let me read what he said. 'The failure of Dr. Schmidt to make a diagnosis of a spinal tumor was not a deviation from the standard of care.' Do you recall that?"

I did.

"Do you disagree with that opinion?"

"No."

"Do you agree with it?"

"Yes."

The defense had also called two other experts, a neurologist named Paul Christman and a neuropathologist named Stonseifer. Had I read their depositions?

I had.

"Do you disagree with any of their opinions?"

"No." They had been asked the same question Harder had been asked and had given the same answer.

"So you agree that Dr. Schmidt's failure to make a diagnosis of a spinal cord tumor was not negligence."

"I never said it was."

"Reporter, please certify that answer. This witness has just contradicted himself."

Schmidt was smiling. He was triumphant. Vindicated.

Angsman turned to the Thompsons' attorney, a woman named Phios. "Patricia, your case is over. Your witness admitted there was no negligence and impeached himself."

"No, I didn't," I said.

"The hell you didn't. You testified that Dr. Schmidt here was negligent in not making the diagnosis. Ongoing negligence you called it."

"I never said that."

"You're a damned liar," he said.

I tried very hard to keep my cool. It was not easy.

"You, sir, are an incompetent listener. I never said that Dr. Schmidt screwed up because he didn't make the diagnosis. I said he screwed up because he never *tried* to make the diagnosis. He never even looked. That was his mistake. Had he looked, he would have made the diagnosis. But he never looked. And not looking is a fundamental error. Even a first-year resident would know that much — a not-very-good first-year resident."

"Dr. Harder never said that."

"No, he didn't."

"Nor did Dr. Christman."

"No."

"Nor Dr. Stonseifer."

"No."

"Why do you think that is?"

"Because they were never asked."

The smile faded from Angsman's face.

"But they will be at trial," Ms. Phios said. "You can bet on that."

"But I never had to make that diagnosis," Schmidt said. "I wasn't wrong not to make the diagnosis. I wasn't negligent. I . . . ." Angsman put his hand on Schmidt's shoulder. He understood, even if his client didn't. He might not have been a competent listener, but he was educable.

The case never came to trial. Schmidt's insurance company settled for the amount of his policy — one million dollars.

Tom Thompson remains in a wheelchair, and his only use for a condom is as a catchall for his urine. He did go to work for Don Paul and is doing very well. Schmidt is still practicing neurology and remains convinced that he did nothing wrong. I ran into Paul Christman at a meeting. He brought up the case. Angsman had called him and asked him the right question. He had given the same answer I gave. So had Stonseifer and Harder.

To get the right answers, you have to ask the right questions. And to make the right diagnosis, you have to do the right tests. If you don't look in the right place, you can't find out what's wrong with the patient. As Abe Baker taught me on the first day of my residency.

CHAPTER FOUR

Epilepsy and the Murder of Lee Harvey Oswald

Who but a guilty man would hire Melvin Belli?

— The author's mother, 1964

Lee Harvey Oswald was shot and killed before my very eyes, in my living room, on my own TV set. And he was simultaneously shot and killed, live, in the living rooms, family rooms, and bedrooms of millions of other Americans, on an otherwise peaceful Sunday morning. There he was, being led, handcuffed, from his cell in the Dallas police lockup through a crowd of reporters, cameramen, and onlookers. And then some overweight guy in a dark suit and a porkpie hat pushed out of the crowd, pulled a gun out of his pocket, and shot Lee Harvey Oswald. It was not a delayed broadcast, or a news clip, or an instant replay. It was live. Instantaneous. And Lee Harvey Oswald, the man who less than forty-eight hours before had shot and killed President John F. Kennedy, was dead. That much I knew the instant I saw them pick up the stretcher and watched Oswald's unsupported head drop down precipitously.

Lee Harvey Oswald was dead. I had seen him shot. Murdered by a man named Jack Ruby. Ruby was an ex-Chicagoan. A punk. A hoodlum. One of those fringe mob-type characters who might have seemed more appropriate in the cast of a local production of *Guys and Dolls* than on the evening news. Even as a hoodlum, success had evaded him. Had he put in the same time and effort on some nonnefarious activity or other, he would have most likely made a far greater success out of his life. But success was not for Jack Ruby.

I paid no attention at all to the Ruby trial. Why should I have? I knew he was guilty. So did every other American who owned a TV. And, as Mother said, if that were not sufficient proof of his guilt, he hired Melvin Belli as his defense attorney. "Who but a guilty man," my mother argued, "would hire Melvin Belli?"

I halfheartedly listened to the news and followed the headlines.

Ruby was tried. Ruby was found guilty. Stories of conspiracies flourished. Somehow they rarely seemed to involve organized crime. Was that too devoid of romance?

Belli withdrew from the case. Elmer Gertz, a civil rights lawyer from Chicago, became Ruby's lawyer. He appealed the verdict. The appeal was upheld and that only generated more theories of further conspiracies.

There would have to be a second trial. But Ruby developed cancer and his cancer spread rapidly and killed him before there was time for his retrial.

That's all I can remember of the sequence. I'm not sure I ever knew very much more. As this was going on, I completed my first year of training in neurology, entered the army for a two-year stint as a neurologist, and wound up spending my last six months of army duty as a neurologist at the 106th Field Hospital in Yokohama, Japan. Professionally, the highlight of that six months was a four-day period when Francis M. Forster, the chairman of the Department of Neurology at the University of Wisconsin and the air force's consultant in neurology, came to Japan in order to look over the neurology facilities and, at the same time, to see some problem patients and present teaching rounds at the various hospitals. One day, he came down to Yokohama to visit the 106th Field Hospital. I presented several patients to him and he made diagnoses on them that I had not even considered. That night he and I and several other neurologists all went to dinner together in Yokohama's Chinatown. After dinner he regaled us with numerous stories from his life in neurology. Today I remember only one of them. Frank Forster told us that he had been a witness at the trial of Jack Ruby, an expert witness for the prosecution.

We were all ears.

Melvin Belli, it seems, held a press conference as soon as he arrived in Dallas to defend Ruby. The press conference had been on TV. I had not watched it. I already knew Ruby was guilty. My mother, I was certain, had been absolutely correct. Belli maintained that his client, poor misunderstood Jack Ruby, had not intentionally murdered anyone. True, he had held the gun that killed Oswald, but he had not intentionally pulled the trigger. Ruby had had an involuntary convulsive jerk that had caused the gun to fire.

A convulsive jerk — a seizure.

What a preposterous notion! A seizure can do many things. But not what I had seen on TV that Sunday morning. No way. But believing that and proving it beyond a benefit of a doubt were two different things.

Frank Forster had watched that news conference and he, too, was skeptical but thought little more of it. Madison was a long way from Dallas, but not as far as he thought. Several days later, Frank received a long-distance phone call from a William Alexander, an assistant D.A. in Dallas. Alexander wanted to know if Professor Forster would review the EEG of a particular individual involved in a criminal proceeding. It didn't take much imagination to figure out just whose EEG that was.

Frank was interested. Who wouldn't have been? But he felt that he had to clear his involvement with the university. The dean of the medical school, Dr. Philip Cohen, felt it was an honor for Frank to have been called. The president of the university, Fred Harvey Harrington, agreed but reminded Frank that he was not representing the University of Wisconsin. In other words, he was on his own if anything went awry.

Frank was also well aware of his own prejudices. He knew Ruby was guilty, and he also had a strong bias against the idea that Ruby had epilepsy. This was based not only on the events of the murder itself, but on the trouble that Belli's statements had already stirred up. Frank spent much of his life treating epileptics. Epilepsy was his main field of interest. In the hysterical aftermath of the assassinations, epileptic patients were being looked upon with increasing suspicion. Much of the slow progress that had been made in changing society's prejudices toward epileptics was being threatened. Frank was worried that if Ruby was shown to have epilepsy, the all-too-common aversion toward epileptics would become worse than ever.

There were, of course, two separate issues to be faced. First, did Jack Ruby have epilepsy? All the term *epilepsy* means is that the afflicted individual has a tendency to have recurrent seizures — episodes of altered behavior caused by abnormal electrical discharges of the brain. Second, and more importantly, if Ruby did indeed have this tendency toward seizures, had he had a seizure that caused his gun to go off?

An EEG might help to answer the first question and even perhaps the second. In general, whether or not a particular episode of behavior in the past was epileptic or not cannot be proved by EEG. All an EEG can do, in most instances, is show whether or not abnormal electrical discharges of the type usually seen in epileptics are present. Whether a particular event in the past was a seizure is a clinical diagnosis based on the history and characteristics of the event. Even if Jack Ruby's EEG demonstrated that he had abnormal discharges of the type associated with epilepsy, it would not prove that the apparently willful behavior we all observed was due to a seizure, Melvin Belli notwithstanding.

I, like other neurologists, was well aware of this problem. We face it every day. Should a seizure patient who is seizure-free and has been seizure-free long enough to legally drive a car wear some type of medical alert bracelet? You might think that he should in order to protect himself. I once had such a patient who was involved in an auto accident. He was driving when another car ran a red light, slammed into his car, and knocked him unconscious. By the time the police arrived, several witnesses had read his bracelet and recalled seeing him shake convulsively and cause the accident. Fortunately, the other driver was honest enough to admit running the red light. After all, not everything that an epileptic does is caused by a seizure. In fact, most activities are not.

Did Ruby have epilepsy?

Had he shot Oswald during one of his seizures?

Frank agreed to review the EEGs.

But when he called Bill Alexander back, Frank asked him to

bring an indeterminate number of records run on the same equipment. In this way, he would not know which was Ruby's EEG. This "blind" technique would preserve his own sense of neutrality. If Ruby was indeed epileptic, it would be taken into account. And then the question would have to be decided whether the murder could have been carried out during a seizure.

Bill Alexander brought a number of EEGs to Madison and met Frank in the library of the Department of Neurology. The EEGs were brought in to Frank one at a time with the title page covered. Frank studied each record carefully. Then he wrote a careful description and interpretation of each record. The record was then removed and a subsequent tracing brought in. He had no idea how many records there were and could not know when he read Jack Ruby's. After the fifth tracing had been interpreted, Bill Alexander said, "That's all. By the way, which do you think is Ruby's?" Frank replied that he could not tell. One record was completely normal, two showed mild slow-wave abnormalities, which were nonspecific, and two were epileptic. He doubted the two with slow-wave abnormalities were Ruby's because they appeared to be identical, and as far as he knew, Ruby was reported to have had a single EEG. Bill Alexander informed him that those two were Ruby's. He hadn't told him previously that there were two EEGs on Ruby. So in this way Frank Forster had preserved the double-blind technique that he cherished. And needless to say, he was delighted that the epileptic records were not Ruby's!

For the trial itself, the Dallas D.A.'s office had a panel of epilepsy/EEG experts. This included Earl Walker of Johns Hopkins, Robert Schwab of Massachusetts General, and one of my old professors, Dr. Roland MacKay of the University of Illinois, in addition to Frank Forster.

They all said the same thing. The EEGs of Jack Ruby demonstrated no abnormal discharges of the type seen in epilepsy. No epilepsy. No seizures.

Who, I wondered, had testified for the defendant? For Jack Ruby and Melvin Belli?

I never had to ask.

Frank merely mentioned that all four of the experts who appeared for the prosecution met after the trial was over and reviewed their individual appraisals of Jack Ruby's EEGs. All of them had noted the same insignificant degree of slow activity. All four had found no evidence of epilepsy. All four had felt that everything else was normal, including the short bursts of 6-per-second rhythmic activity from the temporal lobe, the so-called psychomotor variant. I immediately knew the name of the other expert. The man who had discovered the 6-per-second psychomotor variant. Fred Gibbs had testified for Jack Ruby.

Fred Gibbs is one of the great names in the history of the EEG. He had been in on it almost from the beginning, when Boston City Hospital set up the first EEG lab in the U.S. He'd gone straight from Johns Hopkins Medical School to the EEG lab and rarely emerged. He had never even bothered to take an internship. EEG became his entire professional life. That was his strength and his weakness. He had probably read more EEGs than anyone else in the world. He was the first electroencephalographer to perform systematic studies of EEGs in patients with epilepsy. In the late thirties and early forties, he published a series of classic papers relating specific types of epilepsy to particular wave forms. Petit mal seizures were accompanied by 3-per-second spike-and-wave discharge, grand mal by rapid, generalized high-voltage spikes, temporal lobe or psychomotor seizures by 6-per-second waves in the temporal lobes. And so forth. Each seizure had its own discharge. And each discharge its own seizure. If only the world were that simple.

To Gibbs, it was. To him, epilepsy was an EEG phenomenon, not a clinical one. If the wave was there, the patient had epilepsy. And he had more experience with EEGs than anyone else.

To almost everyone else, the diagnosis of epilepsy was a clinical issue. It depended primarily on the patient's history. Was the history that of a true seizure? The EEG did not make the diagnosis. It helped to define the type of brain wave abnormality associated with a particular historic event. It helped confirm a diagnosis, but it didn't tell you if a patient had a seizure unless he happened to have one during the EEG.

It was a lesson I had learned the hard way. I had spent my first year and a half in the army, as the sole neurologist at Fort Belvoir, just outside Washington, D.C. Much of my time was spent caring for dependents — family members of active-duty G.I.'s. I set up a seizure clinic, the first one in the Washington area. One day, I saw an eight-year-old boy with what clinically seemed to be a true petit mal, brief staring spells lasting a few seconds, but occurring hundreds of times a day. The EEG showed just what Fred Gibbs had originally described, 3-per-second spike-and-wave discharges. Classic petit mal. His seizures were impossible to control. Nothing I did helped for more than a week or two.

Then one day his mother brought his twin brother in with him. A twin brother. An identical twin! Petit mal is hereditary. His twin had to have it, too. I watched him like a hawk. My patient had eight spells during the fifteen-minute visit. His twin, none.

"Is it hereditary?" the mother asked.

"Yes," I said.

"Will my other son get it?"

"Let's do an EEG," I suggested.

So we did. And the twin had spike-and-waves. The same as my patient. In fact, his EEG was worse; his had more abnormal discharges. But he had no spells. None at all. No seizures. Not then. Or any time over the next year that I followed him.

An abnormal EEG does not a diagnosis make.

But to Gibbs, it always did. And nowhere was the discrepancy between Gibbs and most other electroencephalographers and neurologists more marked than in the area of psychomotor variant.

Following his initial work at Boston City Hospital, Gibbs moved to the University of Illinois. There he continued to spend his life in the EEG lab until he finally retired a decade or so ago.

He was not a neurologist. He had never taken a neurology residency. He did not treat patients. As far as I knew, in the time I was there as a student, and later as a resident, Gibbs never saw a patient. Never took a history. All he did was look at brain waves and relate the wave forms to the behavior that others had documented. It was rumored when I was in medical school at the University of Illinois that he wasn't even licensed to practice medicine in Illinois. That was not surprising. Licensure in Illinois requires a completed internship.

The world of electroencephalography had moved on following Gibbs's landmark studies. Wave form was not the entire ball game.

Other factors assumed more importance. Localization, the exact site from which any abnormal discharge emanates. Symmetry of the two sides. These became the issues.

Gibbs continued to describe new specific wave-form abnormalities:

Fourteen- and 6-per-second spikes.

Psychomotor variant.

Right-handed mittens.

Left-handed mittens.

To the rest of the world, these were interesting phenomena in search of significance. To Gibbs, they were the diagnoses. The appearance of one brief episode of a psychomotor variant discharge meant to him the patient had epilepsy.

Any patient.

Jack Ruby.

And the jump from there to Ruby having shot Oswald because of a seizure was one small step. More like a leap of faith.

That had been Gibbs's testimony.

Cross-examination had dwelled on his lack of clinical experience.

"Doctor, when were you graduated from medical school?"

"In 1929."

"Now, where did you intern?"

"I did not intern."

"And where did you have your residency?"

"I did not have a residency."

"When did you become licensed to practice?"

"In 1957."

"Then, Doctor, between 1929 and 1957, you could not treat patients, could you?"

"I treated patients at the Boston City Hospital and the Boston Psychiatric Hospital, and when I came to the University of Illinois, I treated them at the University of Illinois Hospital."

"Doctor, when you set up your own office, you had to have someone else write your prescriptions for you, didn't you?"

"I didn't write prescriptions in my own office."

"Who wrote your prescriptions?"

"I didn't use prescriptions."

"And you didn't treat patients either, did you?"

"Not in my own office."

"No, sir, because you weren't licensed in Illinois. Now, Doctor, of what boards are you a member?"

"I'm not a member of any of the major specialty boards."

"You're not a member of the American Board of Psychiatry?"

"I am not."

"Nor the American Board of Neurology?"

"No."

And his total reliance on EEG. After all, Gibbs had never seen Jack Ruby or taken a history from him. He had based his diagnosis entirely upon his interpretation of the EEGs. And that was where the district attorney attacked. ". . . you agree that the EEG is merely a diagnostic aid, do you not?"

"Well, I know of no other way of making a diagnosis of psychomotor variant epilepsy, and I consider a laboratory test of this sort, having been validated as it has been in this instance, more reliable than a clinical diagnosis. Of course, I think it would be desirable to supplement this laboratory diagnosis with a clinical diagnosis."

"In other words, if I understand you, you say that the EEG is of more value than the clinical diagnosis?"

"I say so most emphatically."

"And if there were a difference in the results between the EEG and the clinical diagnosis, you would prefer to rely upon the EEG?"

"Yes."

This was a position that few if any other experts would have supported. Gibbs had put himself out on a rather lonely limb.

But he was still a potent witness. He had virtually invented the use of EEG in epilepsy. It was up to the experts for the state to cut off that limb. Frank was one of those experts. And Gibbs had trained Frank Forster in EEG. Frank had even coauthored a paper with Gibbs. Frank's testimony itself was quite straightforward. The D.A. asked him the key questions. "Let me ask you, Doctor, considering these two EEGs by themselves, assuming normal neurological tests, normal blood serology, normal spinal puncture, normal head X rays and body X rays, would those EEGs support a diagnosis of any type of epilepsy or psychomotor epilepsy?"

"They would not," Frank replied.

"Doctor, let me ask you a hypothetical question. I'll have to try to include everything in this, but suppose a person were standing on the edge of a crowd, had to make his way through at least one line of the crowd in order to draw a gun and shoot a moving man who was some ten feet away when he first saw him, was a — made some explanation as, 'You rat SOB, you shot the president' or 'You SOB,' was immediately apprehended and within two minutes said something to the effect, 'I intend to kill him,' or — either that or, 'I hope the SOB dies . . . ,' and then, within three minutes of the shooting, said, 'I thought I could get off three shots, but you guys stopped me,' or words to that effect. I'll ask you if, in your opinion, that person could have been suffering psychomotor epilepsy at the time that he did the shooting?"

"No."

Belli then tried to use Forster to credit Gibbs and at the same time use Gibbs to discredit Frank.

"Who has done the most work on psychomotor variants?" Belli asked him.

"Well, one is Dr. Frederick Gibbs in Chicago."

Had Frank read Gibbs's report on Ruby's EEGs?

He had.

"Do you agree or disagree with that report?"

"I disagree."

"You disagree with the report of the man who knows the most about this of anyone in the world? Is that correct?"

"He's assuming something that's not in evidence, Your Honor," the D.A. objected.

"You have already told us this man knows more about psychomotor epilepsy than anyone in the world, haven't you?" Belli continued, looking at Frank Forster and intentionally quoting him not quite correctly.

"I said he was the one that had done the most work on it," Frank replied, correcting Belli's misquote.

"But didn't you say that he is the man that knows more about this than anyone in the world?" Belli insisted.

"Dr. Gibbs has done the most work on this. These are his findings. They are not completely accepted by the profession," Frank calmly replied.

Belli also hit on Frank's relationship to Gibbs. How could Frank disagree with his teacher? The man who had taught him how to interpret EEGs?

"Because," Frank answered, "in this instance, he is wrong."

The jury agreed with Frank and the other experts who testified for the prosecution.

Jack Ruby had never been very lucky. And he wasn't lucky in his timing. Had his trial taken place ten years earlier, it might have turned out differently. That had happened in at least one jurisdiction shortly after Gibbs had published his original data on 14- and 6-per-second positive spikes, another of the "abnormal" discharges he invented. No one else had paid much attention to these normal variants. His was the only data that existed. The only game in town. Attacks of rage, he claimed, occurred in 15 percent of those patients with 14- and 6-per-second positive spikes in the EEG. Out of 427 patients with these positive spikes, 45 had a history of rage attacks and 4 committed murder during an attack.

It was a defense that worked for Rose Valenti. She was forty-seven years old and for nearly thirty years had been married to a husband who often abused her. One day he threatened to kill her and knocked her unconscious. That night, when he was sleeping, she shot him five times and killed him. She claimed that she had no memory at all of her act.

An EEG was performed fifty-four days later. During sleep, it contained 6- and 14-per-second positive spikes. The judge concluded his long instructions to the jury as follows:

> "If it appears from the evidence that the mind of the accused at the time of the commission of the act charged, was in a diseased and unsound state, and that the disease existed to a degree that for the time being it overwhelmed the reason and

judgment and obliterated the will to such an extent as to cause her to act without being conscious of the act itself, again the act was not that of a voluntary agent, but was the involuntary act of the body without the concurrence of the mind directing it, and the person named cannot be held responsible."

Rose Valenti was found innocent.

Today Fred Gibbs is retired. No one has picked up his mantle. In all probability there would be no one to testify for Melvin Belli were his case to come up again. And, hopefully, Rose Valenti wouldn't even be tried. Epilepsy had nothing to do with her lack of guilt.

AUTHOR'S NOTE

The medical testimony from the trial of Jack Ruby is a matter of public record. It is more accessible than most trial transcripts in that it was published in a medical journal, *Trauma*, in December 1964. This essay is drawn, in part, from those transcripts as well as from my recollections of Frank Forster's telling of the tale in 1966 and Frank's own written memoirs. When I called Frank, who is now retired, to discuss this case with him, he informed me that he was writing his autobiography and that he had written a chapter on his medical-legal experience. He was kind enough to send this on to me. Frank was also kind enough to read this and correct some errors. If any slipped through, the fault is mine.

CHAPTER FIVE

Just Dandy

Serious sport has nothing to do with fair play. It is bound up with hatred, jealousy, boastfulness and disregard of all the rules.

— George Orwell
Shooting an Elephant

In 1988, I was reviewing a medical malpractice case on behalf of one of the doctors who was being sued. The issues had to do with the need to perform a CT scan in order to properly evaluate a patient being seen in an E.R. following minor head trauma. The expert for the plaintiff had testified in his deposition that the failure of the E.R. physician to get a CT scan was a deviation from the standard of care, definite malpractice. The expert was a plastic surgeon who had at one time been an E.R. physician. He had further testified at his deposition that his authority for his opinion was the chapter on head trauma in a famous surgery textbook written by Walter Dandy. I read this statement and knew that the case was over.

The first CT scans were done in 1973. Walter Dandy was one of the great figures in the history of neurosurgery. He had been called in to evaluate George Gershwin for Gershwin's terminal brain tumor. I had a profound respect for Dandy and his accomplishments, even his opinions. Walter Dandy had, however, died in 1946. That made it most unlikely that he had written very much on CT scans. I also believed that it had been reasonable for the E.R. physician not to order a CT scan. I said that at my deposition. But we never said a word about Walter Dandy.

I had told the defense attorneys all about the very late Walter

Dandy. But they never even broached the subject at the deposition. They had far bigger and far more dramatic plans. The lawyers wanted to impeach the other side's expert in court. On the record. And destroy him once and for all. He was a hired gun who testified in twenty to thirty cases a year. And he testified about everything. Always for plaintiff and always for big bucks.

And they did just that.

At the trial, the plastic surgeon testified that the failure to get a CT scan was malpractice and that he depended on Walter Dandy for this opinion.

Walter Dandy, the famous neurosurgeon from Johns Hopkins? he was asked.

Yes.

Did he know the year that the first CT scans were performed in the U.S.?

No, not offhand.

Would he accept 1973?

He would. That seemed about right to him.

"And you know about the use of CT scans in evaluating patients who have been in accidents because of Walter Dandy. He's the real authority on CT scans in brain injury. Correct?"

"In brain injury. Yes, sir!"

"And how, pray tell, did you learn exactly what Walter Dandy's opinions of CT scans were?"

"I . . ." the witness began.

"Was it a séance? Or did you use a Ouija board?"

The plaintiff's attorney started to object. "Judge, he is badgering my witness. And making a mockery of his testimony. I request that you instruct the jury to disregard his last question."

"Judge," the defense attorney said, "I would like this document identified. It is a copy of the death certificate of Dr. Walter Dandy. He died in 1946. The first CT scans were done twenty-seven years later. I was just trying to discover how the witness learned Dr. Dandy's thoughts about the use of CT scans. Séances and Ouija boards seemed reasonable possibilities. I wonder if the witness has any other explanation."

He didn't.

The plaintiff's case was blown. I never even testified. The plaintiff settled for a few bucks, a nuisance settlement that represented less than the cost of continuing the trial.

That's how the game is played.

To WIN.

If that plastic surgeon ever appears in court again, he can be asked about his testimony in this case. An expert's previous "expert" activities are an appropriate avenue of inquiry. This impeachment would cast doubt on any authorities he ever used and any opinions he might form.

And he, have no doubt about it, will hear about the late Walter Dandy every time he walks into court.

Why?

Because winning is the only thing.

CHAPTER SIX

Taking a Risk

A rule of thumb in the matter of medical advice is to take
everything any doctor says with a grain of aspirin.

— Goodman Ace

The weeks between Thanksgiving and Christmas were always
the busiest weeks in Jane Shannon's life. No sooner had she cleaned
the house after Thanksgiving dinner for thirty or more assorted
guests, including all eight grandchildren, than the real rush started.
Getting the house ready for Christmas. Christmas shopping. Re-
hearsals for the Christmas choir program at St. Paul's Church.
Working part-time at her son's women's clothing store during his
busiest season. Volunteer work. Putting dinner on the table each
night for her and John; she couldn't neglect John. Babysitting for
the grandchildren. And so much more. She should never have
allowed Father Timothy O'Connor to talk her into making an
appointment with a new doctor. Just because she had mentioned
that she hadn't seen a doctor in twenty-seven years, since John,
Junior, had been born. She might be sixty-two, but she was in
perfect health. But Bridget Riley had just died of . . . He had not
said the word. She knew what Bridget had died of. Cancer of the
womb. Bridget Riley also hadn't seen a doctor in decades. They
can find those things, Father O'Connor told her, before they're
bad enough to kill you.

Jane didn't like the idea of some doctor probing inside her body.
It didn't seem right to her. Had the Virgin Mary had to go through
such indignities? She was glad she hadn't asked the Father that. He
was too young to understand women like her.

Still, he had insisted.

Why hadn't he just asked her to do a penance or two? More

volunteer work? Help cook and serve Christmas dinner at the parish? That was all old Father Mack ever did. May Jesus bless his soul.

Father Timothy O'Connor was adamant.

Jane Shannon relented. What other choice did she have?

On December tenth, she saw Dr. James Scanlon. He had been poor Bridget's doctor. He'd done whatever he could for her, poor soul. He was only thirty-four-or-five years old, a mere child, but he seemed nice enough. And thorough. Too thorough. He probed her everywhere. And listened all over her body. And pushed and felt everything. And did tests. Blood tests. A chest X ray. And an EKG.

And then he sat down to tell her the results. He had found two problems.

The way he said "problems" worried Jane. She didn't think she had any problems at all. And he said she had two. Bridget had only had one.

Her blood pressure was too high.

Someone had told her that once before, she recalled.

When?

She thought hard. Twenty years ago. She'd been in an auto accident and struck her head. They'd made her go to some emergency room. The nurse there had taken her blood pressure and said it was above normal.

Dr. Scanlon wrote that on her record.

"It's probably been elevated all these years," he said.

"How can you tell?" she asked.

"It shows on your heart tracing."

"Oh." She nodded.

He told her she would have to take some medicine. He gave her a prescription for something he called a water pill. It would make her go to the bathroom more often. And she would have to watch how much salt she ate. She would have to cook with less salt. He gave her a list of typed instructions. Cooking instructions, no less. What was he? Some sort of a chef?

So much for the first problem.

Jane smiled at Dr. Scanlon. She gazed at the sheet and dutifully folded it and put it and the prescription into her purse. John liked salt on his food. He liked the way her food tasted. So did she. She had lived with her high blood pressure for twenty years. She could live with it another twenty years.

And the one thing she wouldn't take was a water pill. Some of her friends had taken them. She had had five children. Her bladder was weak. She dribbled at times. The very last thing she needed was more water in her bladder. Didn't young doctors understand such problems? He had probed her down there. Didn't he realize?

On to problem two.

She had a bruit.

A what?

A murmur. A noise.

Where?

In her neck.

What did that mean?

That the blood vessels going to her brain, from her heart to the brain, might be blocked up.

This, she realized, might be serious.

It could cause a stroke.

That scared her more than Bridget's troubles had. Her dad had had a stroke. For five years she had nursed him. He had been unable to move his right arm and leg. Unable to speak. He couldn't even go to church.

That was the last thing she wanted to have happen to her. The very last thing. "Sweet Jesus," she prayed softly.

She needed a test, the doctor told her.

Whatever she needed, she would do; but couldn't it wait until after Christmas?

No.

Why not?

She could have that stroke any minute.

"Blessed Mary, Mother of God." She repeated that twice.

The test she got was called an ultrasound test. She had seen Dr. Scanlon on Thursday. She went to Holy Trinity Community Hospital on Monday for the test. The test took about an hour. A young doctor named Donovan did it. He just kept rubbing something that looked like a cross between a microphone and a small flashlight over her neck and mumbling to himself. When he was done rubbing and mumbling, he said he would send her results to Dr. Scanlon the next day.

That was fine. She had an appointment to see him on Thursday.

As soon as she walked into Dr. Scanlon's office, Jane knew that he had the results of her test and that the news was not good.

Before he'd let her know what they were, he once again listened to her neck. The bruits were still there, he informed her.

Then he checked her high blood pressure. It was not quite as high. Still too high, but better. Closer to normal. The medicine was helping. They would give it another few weeks before deciding if she needed something stronger.

Jane said nothing. The unfilled prescription was still in her purse.

"The test?" she asked.

Dr. Scanlon shook his head gravely. "You have blockage of both of the big arteries in your neck. Critical blockage."

She didn't know precisely what "critical blockage" meant, but she could tell by the way he said it that it was bad.

"You need another test."

She listened as Dr. Scanlon told her about the angiogram he felt she needed. It was basically an X ray, but this X ray had to be done in the hospital.

What hospital?

Holy Trinity.

It would be done by Dr. Ruiz, a radiologist who specialized in such X rays. He would put a needle into her groin.

But the problem was in her neck.

Scanlon smiled.

The needle would then be threaded up the big arteries of her body until it was near her neck. Then Dr. Ruiz would inject a dye and take some X rays and see those blocked arteries in her neck. Then they'd know exactly what they had to do to keep her from having a stroke.

She didn't want to have a stroke.

Of course not. She told Scanlon about her father.

"I want you to go into the hospital on Sunday. Dr. Ruiz will do the angiogram on Monday. I will see you again next Tuesday."

"But next Friday is Christmas. I have so much to do. At home. For the church, the choir, my son's store . . ."

"If we don't do the right thing, you could have a stroke before Christmas. You have critical stenosis on both sides. Critical."

Jane was now truly frightened. She'd do almost anything to prevent having a stroke. Maybe even undergo surgery. The thought of someone cutting into her body frightened her. That's what had killed her mother. A routine hysterectomy, the doctor had said. She had a tired womb. A simple operation. Nothing to worry about. Her mother had died on the operating room table.

No. She didn't want an operation. Anything but surgery.

On Sunday, December 20, she checked into Holy Trinity Community Hospital. She expected to see Dr. Scanlon. And to meet Dr. Ruiz. But that wasn't what happened.

Some young doctor with an Indian name took her history and examined her. Sort of. He never even listened to her neck.

Didn't he care about her bruits? That was why she was in the hospital. Critical stenosis. Whatever that meant.

Another young doctor also came into the room. He was an Asian of some sort. Korean or something. And spoke very poor English. All she could tell from what he said was that he worked with Dr. Ruiz. He told her they would do an angiogram. She had to sign something.

She signed.

Were there any dangers? she asked.

"No. We do all time. Every day. No problems. A simple test."

He, too, did not listen to her neck.

The next morning, she had the angiogram, the simple test they had all told her about. She hardly felt anything as Dr. Ruiz put the needle into her groin. About ten minutes later they told her to hold still for the X ray.

Suddenly she felt a blast of heat shoot through her neck and into her head. It was like an explosion. Like hot oil burning its way through her head.

Like the fires of hell.

Straight into her eyes.

And then it was gone.

"All done," the Korean said. "No so bad. Like I tell to you."

Three hours later, they sent her home.

On Tuesday, she saw Dr. Scanlon once again. It was much like her previous visit. Her blood pressure was still too high to suit him. And the noises were still there in her neck. The angiogram had shown the same thing that the first study had shown. The ultra-sound. "Both of your big arteries in the neck," he informed her, "are blocked up." This she already knew. But then Dr. Scanlon went on to explain what it all meant. These arteries were called the carotid arteries. Those were what kept her both alive and healthy. They supplied most of the blood to the brain. And she had bad blocks on both sides. Both carotid arteries. Severe stenosis.

"Critical stenosis."

That same word again. "Critical."

If they didn't do something, her brain would not get enough blood and she would have a stroke.

Wasn't there anything they could do?

Surgery.

Was there anything else? She hated the idea of any kind of surgery. It frightened her. Her mother . . .

No. She needed surgery.

But her mother.

And her father, Dr. Scanlon reminded her. She didn't want to have a stroke and end up like her father, did she? A helpless invalid. Unable to go to church. To Mass. To . . .

No. Anything but that.

Surgery was the answer. She should see Dr. Fredericks. He was their vascular surgeon. He did these operations all the time. Every week. Every day almost.

She could see him after Christmas, she suggested.

"Tomorrow," Dr. Scanlon said, "at one in the afternoon. I already called him and he said he could squeeze you in."

"But I have so much to do."

"And if you have your stroke while you're waiting to see the doctor, what then?"

What choice did she have? Very little. From what they were saying, it was either surgery or a stroke.

John went with her to see Dr. Fredericks. Neither of them had ever seen an office quite like it. There was even a fountain in the waiting room. And the doctor didn't wear a white coat. He wore a sports jacket.

He didn't take any history from her. He had a summary from Dr. Scanlon.

"No symptoms," he commented.

She didn't understand.

"Your bad vessels haven't caused you any problems yet. No weakness. No dizziness."

No, she agreed. They hadn't.

"Yet," he said.

It was the way he said "yet" that scared her.

He listened to her neck and frowned. He seemed very concerned by what he heard. He then went over to the wall and flicked a switch on an X-ray view box. The light came on. There were X rays already in place. Dr. Fredericks looked at them, shook his head, and mumbled to himself.

"Come over here," he said.

Jane and John both came over to the view box.

"This is your angiogram," Dr. Fredericks announced. "And here's what's wrong." With that, he pointed out the white columns that were her carotid arteries and the dark areas of narrowing that were the blockage.

"Right carotid artery," he said. "Seventy percent stenosis.

"Left carotid, eighty percent.

"Critical stenosis."

That same phrase. It still scared her.

"You need surgery."

"Isn't there anything else you can do?" John asked.

"No."

"No medicines?"

"No. If I don't do the surgery and remove those blocks," he said, "your wife will have a stroke."

"We know she might."

"Not might," he said. "Will. If I don't operate on her and take away those blocks, she will have a stroke."

"Are you sure of that?"

"One hundred percent. There is no question about that. She has critical stenosis."

"When will she have the stroke?"

"Who can tell? Today. Tonight. Tomorrow. It certainly could be tomorrow."

"Then we shouldn't wait," John concluded.

"Of course not. I've already made arrangements." The doctor turned to Jane. "I have put you on the operating room schedule for tomorrow at eight in the morning. You will go into the hospital this afternoon."

"But tomorrow is Christmas Eve. I sing with the choir. I have to be home with my family."

"They can sing without you."

"Can't it wait?"

"You could have a stroke tomorrow unless I operate and open up those arteries and save your brain. And you don't want to have a stroke, do you?" He would operate on the left carotid artery tomorrow. That was where the blockage was worse. More critical. And the left side of the brain controlled speech. She certainly didn't want to have a stroke that caused her to lose the ability to speak.

She didn't.

He would do the other side right after Christmas. She would be home just after New Year's Day.

As she walked to the door, she remembered a question. "Are there any risks?"

"The real risk is you walking around with those critically blocked arteries. Let me worry about the risks."

Mrs. Shannon was admitted to Holy Trinity Community Hospital at five-thirty in the evening on December twenty-third. Dr. Scanlon stopped by at about seven to say hello and wish her well. He reassured both the Shannons that surgery was the right choice. Dr. Fredericks was very good. He did several of these operations every week. His patients rarely had problems.

While he was still there, a nurse came by. Jane had to sign something.

"What?"

"The consent form for the surgery." The nurse was certain the doctor had told her everything about the surgery.

She signed.

And John signed as one of the witnesses. The nurse also signed it.

At seven-fifteen in the morning, they took Jane Shannon to the operating room.

At seven-forty-five, the anesthesiologist put a needle into her arm, and almost immediately she went to sleep.

By eight o'clock, Dr. Fredericks was already at work. The procedure he was doing was called a left carotid endarterectomy. It consists of removing the block from the left carotid artery.

At eight twenty-five, he placed a tube into the artery, a detour, an alternate route for the blood so that the brain would continue to get the blood it needed. Then he began to remove the area of stenosis itself.

By nine-fifteen he was done. He removed the tube and closed-up the clean artery.

At nine forty-five Jane Shannon was taken from the operating room to the postsurgical recovery area.

At eleven-thirty, Dr. Fredericks came by to see her.

She felt fine.

Her speech was fine.

She could move both arms and legs.

"We'll do the other side on Tuesday," he said.

At twelve-thirty, John came in to see her. He was so happy. Dr. Fredericks had talked to him. Everything had gone well. The surgery had been a complete success. The second operation would be even easier.

"It's tomorrow," he said to his wife, "and you didn't have a stroke. Thanks to Dr. Fredericks."

"And Jesus."

John agreed.

At two-thirty the nurse woke her up to say something to her. Jane couldn't understand the nurse. And when Jane tried to ask the nurse to repeat what she had said, her own words were garbled. Jane tried to lift her right hand. She couldn't. She remembered her dad. She knew what had happened. No doctor had to tell her. It was tomorrow and she had had her stroke.

Jane left the hospital six weeks later. She never went back for her second operation. After all, she never recovered from the first. When she went home, she still had severe weakness on the right side of her body and a severe speech deficit. Right hemiplegia and aphasia. Just like her father. She would never again sing in the choir. Or help her son in the clothing store or cook a Thanksgiving dinner or take care of her grandchildren. It would be their job to help take care of her. To baby-sit for grandma and to try to figure out what she needed when she babbled at them, all but incomprehensibly. Dr. Fredericks told them if he had operated on her sooner, this never would have happened. He had tried, but it had been too late.

A year later, she was still no better. Another Christmas had come and gone. She could walk with assistance, but her right hand was all but useless. And her speech was not really speech at all, more a primitive sort of prelanguage with which she could communicate basic needs, like the need to go to the bathroom, the need for water, pain.

And her family knew she would never get any better.

So did she. That much she understood.

Her husband and son went to see their family lawyer. Jane had to be declared incompetent so that her husband could handle all their affairs. John wanted to sell the house and buy a smaller one, one that he could manage. But their house was owned by both of them jointly. He had talked to a real estate person and she had told him what papers were needed.

The lawyer's name was Murphy. He listened to John tell the entire story. They needed a doctor to say that Jane was not competent to handle her own affairs. Had she seen a doctor in the last year?

No.

She would have to see one.

Who?

It made no difference to Murphy. Why not call Dr. Fredericks?

The next day John did just that.

Dr. Fredericks would not see Jane. There was nothing more he could do for her. No more operations. Nothing. She had had the stroke he was trying to prevent. It wasn't his fault.

His fault? Up until that point, John had never thought that Jane's stroke was anyone's fault. She had had critical stenosis. Whatever that meant.

Fredericks insisted that he had done nothing wrong.

John had never thought he had.

Mrs. Shannon should see Dr. Scanlon.

John called. Scanlon agreed to see her and did. There wasn't much he could do. He put her on some new medicine for her blood pressure. Not a water pill this time, since getting to the bathroom was such a problem. It was called Tenormin. It was what the doctor called a beta-blocker. John had no idea what that meant.

Dr. Scanlon reassured John that Jane had needed the surgery — John knew that. He accepted that — and that no one had done anything wrong. That bad things do happen sometimes. Even to good people. And that the surgery did sometimes cause strokes.

"The surgery caused this?" John asked. That was a notion that he had not put together in his mind. They had done the surgery to prevent a stroke. But Jane had had the stroke. He had thought that the surgery just hadn't worked. That was what Dr. Fredericks had said.

"Yes," Scanlon said. "The surgery caused the stroke. Strokes are a known risk of that operation."

Dr. Fredericks had never told them that. He had lied to them. Had that been his only lie?

"But," Scanlon hastened to add, "Jane needed the surgery. Without it she would have had a stroke."

"Does she still have the other bruit?"

Scanlon hadn't bothered to check. He took out his stethoscope and listened. The bruit was still there.

"Will she have a stroke on the other side?" John asked.

"Of course."

"Fredericks says she can't be operated on."

"Another operation would be much too dangerous," Scanlon agreed.

Of course, John realized suddenly, she had gone a whole year with that other bruit without having another stroke, and she had had "critical stenosis" on that side, too. Or at least that was what Fredericks had told them. Might that have happened on the left side too? Could she have gone a year without her stroke? "Isn't there anything you can do?" He was becoming desperate.

"There is. We can give her medicine."

There was a medicine to prevent strokes? That was news to him. It was probably something new. Like the beta-blocker.

"What?" he asked.

"Aspirin," he was told.

"Aspirin!"

"Yes. One each day. Aspirin can prevent strokes and heart attacks."

How?

No one was certain. But when the arteries get clogged like the ones in Jane's neck, particles called platelets collect on them and then break off and go to the brain and cause a stroke. Aspirin helps prevent that.

John followed what he was saying. That was why doctors took aspirin and not Tylenol. The TV ad. If doctors were going to an island, they'd take aspirin. Not Advil or Tylenol. But not for headaches, but to prevent strokes and heart attacks.

"And last year, couldn't she have taken aspirin? No one ever suggested that she could take aspirin . . . ."

"She needed that surgery, John. You heard what Dr. Fredericks said."

John had. And Fredericks had lied to him at least once.

I first heard about the case from a lawyer named Richard Donovan with whom I had worked a couple of times in the past when he had worked in one of the large Chicago defense firms. He was now out on his own, representing plaintiffs, or as he put it, working the other side of the street. The Shannons had gone back to Murphy and Murphy had sent them on to Donovan, who had called to pick my brain.

Donovan told me the story as John Shannon had told it to him.

"That SOB," I said.

"Who?"

"Fredericks. There was no reason to do the surgery."

"No reason!"

He was surprised by my statement. "If she was my patient, I

would not even have sent her for the angiogram, much less surgery."

"But she had disease. It's on the X rays. Even I can see that on the angiogram."

It was time to step back a couple of steps and start from scratch. Mrs. Shannon had disease. There was no question about that. She had atherosclerosis involving the great vessels in her neck with incomplete blockade of both carotid arteries. The atherosclerosis was the result of the untreated high blood pressure she'd had for so many years.

"So she needed the surgery," Donovan protested.

"Why do you think that?"

"Blocking the arteries going to the brain causes strokes."

"If only it were that simple."

"It isn't?"

"Not at all. In order to know if she needed surgery, you have to know three things. What is the natural history of partially blocked arteries in someone without any symptoms? What are the chances that that patient will have a stroke? That's fact one."

"So tell me."

"We don't know precisely."

"I need precise answers. I'm a poor country lawyer."

Who had been at the top of his class at Northwestern Law School, I thought to myself.

"Rich, let me put it in legal terms. More probably than not, she would never have had a stroke. People with high blood pressure and bad arteries in the neck also have bad arteries elsewhere. They usually die of heart disease before they have a stroke."

"So it doesn't cause strokes."

"I didn't say that. What I said is that such bad arteries are a risk factor for a stroke. They increase the chances of a stroke — the risk. But that risk is still small."

"How small?"

"A couple of percent a year. Maybe ten to fifteen percent in five years."

"I understand."

"Fact two. Does the surgery in such patients alleviate or decrease this risk?"

"That's the key question," he agreed. "It must be very effective to warrant the risk."

"It ought to be."

"Is it?"

"We have no idea at all. The long-term value has never been proved at all. In fact, right now, the federal government, through the National Institutes of Health, is funding a multicenter study all across the country to see if it does any good at all."

"Wow," was his only reply.

"And, of course, the surgery can cause strokes."

That he already knew. "How frequently?"

"In the best of hands, one to two percent. In community hospitals, where they do fewer, the incidence of such complications is often higher." And Holy Trinity was a community hospital.

"So we've got a case," he said triumphantly.

"Why?"

"The surgery was not indicated. That's called surgical mayhem. There was no reason to do it. No one knows if it helps. Doing it was therefore a deviation from the standard of care."

"You're absolutely right, in my opinion."

I could hear him counting the dollars.

"Except for one minor issue."

"What's that?"

"Mine is not the only opinion in this issue. Cardiovascular surgeons do procedures like this all the time. For them it's the standard of care. I can't say that Fredericks's decision to do surgery was anything that deviated from the way cardiovascular surgeons practice medicine. They all do it. Every week."

"But . . ."

"That's why I teach my residents that the decision as to whether or not a patient needs surgery is too important to leave up to the surgeon."

"So . . ."

"There's no case. It's a known risk of a procedure that other surgeons all would have done. They all practice bad medicine in my opinion. Even at my hospital. But there's nothing I can do to stop it."

Rich was no longer counting the dollars. "Thanks. Send me a

bill for the consult. You saved me from wasting my time. I was going to take Fredericks's deposition tomorrow. I'll just withdraw from the case."

"I will."

"I can't believe that Fredericks can lie to his patient and get away with it."

"How did he lie?"

"He told them that unless she had the surgery, she'd have a stroke."

"I doubt that."

"Why? That's what John Shannon told me he said."

"That's what Mr. Shannon remembers. And what patients and their families remember from such conversations is often inaccurate. No honest surgeon could possibly have told them that."

Richard Donovan did not withdraw from the case. Instead, he spent the next day taking a discovery deposition from Dr. Fredericks.

Dr. Fredericks said pretty much what Donovan had expected him to say. Mrs. Shannon had very bad disease in both carotid arteries in her neck. Severe blockage. "Critical stenosis," he called it.

Was he certain of that?

Yes.

How could he be?

The ultrasound studies and the angiograms had both shown a critical degree of blockage.

What could be done to help her?

Surgery.

Nothing else?

No.

Was he certain of that?

Absolutely. When a patient had critical stenosis, only surgery helped. And Mrs. Shannon had critical stenosis, on both sides.

Was he sure that there was no other possible treatment?

He was more than sure; he was adamant.

Had he told her that?

"Her and her husband. I told them both. Nothing else could prevent her from having a stroke. Only I could do that. I'm sure Mr. Shannon remembers what I said."

So was Richard Donovan.

"Why did she need the surgery?"

"Why? That's obvious. Without the surgery, she would have a stroke."

"You mean she might have a stroke?"

"No. No. Not might. Would. If I had done nothing, she would have had a stroke. And she didn't want that," Fredericks said, expanding on his reply. "I'm not some epidemiologist talking about nonsense like risk factors. I'm talking about a real patient. That's just what I told her. Without the surgery, she would have a stroke. No question about it. I told her that. I told her husband."

"So she had critical stenosis."

"Yes."

"So critical that it was an emergency."

"Yes. Yes. You understand."

"And she had critical stenosis on the other side, too, didn't she?"

"Yes. She had very bad disease. Both sides were critical."

"So, she needed operation on both sides."

"Yes."

"To prevent strokes on both sides."

"That is correct."

"Without the surgery on the left carotid, she would have a stroke on the left side of her brain. And without surgery on the right carotid, she would have a stroke on the right side."

"I see you've been studying anatomy."

"I try," Donovan replied. "And you agree?"

"Most certainly."

"And both sides were critical."

Fredericks agreed. They were both emergencies.

Did he operate on the right side?

No.

Had she ever had a stroke there?

He had no idea.

"She hasn't," Donovan informed him. "On which side did you operate?"

"The left side."

"On which side did she have the stroke?"

Fredericks was talking much more softly now. And slowly.
"The left side."

"And what caused that stroke?"

"She had a critical stenosis and . . ."

Donovan interrupted him. "What caused her stroke which occurred within twenty-four hours of your surgery?"

"Strokes are a known complication . . ."

He again interrupted the surgeon. "I didn't ask you that. I asked
you what caused the stroke."

"Do I have to answer that?" Fredericks asked his lawyer.

"If you have an opinion within a reasonable degree of medical
and surgical certainty, you can give it. If you have no opinion, you
can say that," his lawyer informed him.

"Dr. Fredericks, was the stroke caused by the surgery?" Donovan insisted.

Fredericks and his lawyer held a whispered conversation. At the
end of which he asked the reporter to repeat the question, and after
listening, said, "Yes."

"Did you warn her that that might happen?"

"Of course not."

My deposition took place about two years later. Mrs. Shannon was
still no better. She still had severe aphasia and right-sided weakness. She still had a bruit on the right side of her neck. She was still
on aspirin and she still had not had a stroke on the right side of her
brain. I had agreed to act as an expert witness for the plaintiff. In
that role, I was to address three issues. Causation, prognosis, and
the issue of informed consent.

I was to give a discovery deposition. The other side had the
opportunity to ask me questions to discover my opinions. My
opinions on causation and prognosis were very simple. They were
also not being contested. The surgery had caused the stroke. Even
Dr. Fredericks agreed to that. And Mrs. Shannon would never get
any better. She would live out her life severely disabled.

Wasn't a stroke a known risk of such a procedure? Fredericks's
lawyer asked.

It was, I admitted.

So what was the problem?

"He lied to her. He withheld facts. He misled her, and as a result he never obtained a legal informed consent. As far as I'm concerned, what he did was surgical mayhem," I began.

"He lied?"

"Yes."

"Those are strong words."

"Not strong enough."

"And how did he lie to her?"

"Three times," I said.

"Three?"

"Yes. Three lies. First, he told her that without the surgery she would have a stroke. That was untrue. While carotid stenosis that has caused no symptoms may be a risk factor for stroke, not everyone with such stenosis will ever have a stroke. Most, in fact, never do."

I then went on to explain what I had already explained to Richard Donovan. "So," I concluded, "Dr. Fredericks lied when he told Mr. and Mrs. Shannon that she definitely would have a stroke."

"That's your opinion."

"That was the first lie," I replied. "His second lie was telling her that her 'critical stenosis' was an emergency. That she might have a stroke that day. It was not an emergency. She had had the stenosis for years. Her chances of immediately developing a stroke were exceedingly low. It was no emergency. Lie number two."

I stopped. Should I just go on or wait for another question? The lawyer nodded.

"Lie number three. He had told her that if he did the surgery, she *wouldn't* have a stroke. Not true. It is *possible* that asymptomatic stenosis may increase the risk of a stroke and that surgical removal of the stenosis *may* decrease this increased risk, but this is *unproven*. Had he said he thought she needed the surgery, that would have been acceptable. But he didn't; he said she had to have it and that it would prevent her from having a stroke. Three little lies."

"Was that all he did that was wrong?"

"Far from it." He'd asked me an open-ended question, so I gave an open-ended answer. There are three basic elements in an informed consent: disclosure of the major risks of the treatment or procedure being contemplated, an accurate assessment of the benefits that can be reasonably expected, and a discussion of alternative forms of treatment.

"Our good friend Dr. Fredericks omitted a few of these. He lied about the possible benefits of the surgery. The other elements he just omitted. He never discussed any other forms of therapy, including the true prognosis if nothing at all was done." She was now on aspirin, I reminded them, and had not had a stroke on the other side. "And, he never told her that the surgery had the potential of causing a stroke."

"And how, Dr. Klawans, do you really know what he said and didn't say to the patient? Were you there when he discussed the surgery?"

"No, but there was a very reliable witness."

"John Shannon. He is an interested party."

"No. Dr. Fredericks. He said it all in his own deposition."

Hoist with his own petard.

My deposition was over.

Fredericks was ready for a courtroom battle. No neurologist could tell him how to practice medicine. He was right. All of his cardiovascular colleagues did the same thing he did. They all operated on patients with bruits that caused no symptoms. Surgery on carotid stenosis is one of the most commonly performed operations in the U.S. If surgeons told these patients what I said they should, then half the patients wouldn't get the operations they needed.

Dr. Fredericks's insurance company was not willing to risk a trial. They paid the Shannons one and a half million dollars. The hospital also threw in the towel. Their culpability was due to the fact that a nurse had obtained the actual signed consent form. They redid their standard form and mandated that the surgeon himself had to obtain the appropriate signature. They also began to monitor Dr. Fredericks's rate of complications. In 1986, he performed forty-two carotid endarterectomies. Not exactly one every day. Five patients suffered strokes at the time of surgery or immediately thereafter. That complication rate is unacceptable, but the hospital did nothing. In 1987, the rate was 13 percent, eight out of sixty-three. Still they did nothing until two of these eight patients sued. In their suits, they named both Dr. Fredericks and the hospital. He had not warned the patients that the surgery could cause a stroke. The hospital was sued for allowing him to do a procedure with an unacceptably high rate of complications.

Richard Donovan was the lawyer for both of the plaintiffs.

Fredericks no longer operates at Holy Trinity. He still does carotid endarterectomies, but he now does them at another hospital. It's easier. There's no monitoring of his complications, and the nurses will take care of all the small details — like obtaining signed consent forms. All he does is admit the patients and operate on them and keep the beds filled, with his successes and failures.

CHAPTER SEVEN

Better Living Through Chemistry

Everyone is famous for fifteen minutes.

— Andy Warhol

Vic Evers is a lawyer in the central part of Illinois, near St. Louis. Although I had known him for several years, we had never really worked together. We had met when I had been examining plaintiffs involved in a dioxin spill that had occurred in Sturgeon, Missouri. He was one of the lawyers with the firm that represented the plaintiffs. It wasn't his case, per se; he didn't make the big decisions or ask the key questions; but he was around and we kept seeing each other and became friends. We respected each other professionally and reminisced together about old ball players. What more was needed to get through a dinner in a barely acceptable restaurant in downstate Illinois?

Every once in a while Vic called me to ask about a case. Usually, the cases were ones in which I had no interest, so nothing came of his calls. Then one day, he called to tell me a story. He'd been at a reception of some sort and had run into a young man who claimed to be famous.

"Everybody is famous for fifteen minutes," I said.

"Sure," he replied, "but this young man had the article to prove his fame."

I had no interest in some over-aged adolescent who carried his press clippings from the *East St. Louis Daily Bugle* or whatever in his wallet. I don't even keep a copy of the Sunday *New York Times* book section review of *Toscanini's Fumble* in my wallet.

I wasn't even half listening until I heard the phrase, "the *Journal of Pediatrics*."

"What?" I asked.

"Haven't you been listening?"

"Of course I have."

"He had two articles from the *Journal of Pediatrics* with him," Vic repeated. "He never goes anywhere without them."

"Like his American Express card," I suggested.

"He doesn't have one of those. This kid dropped out of high school. He works as a window washer."

By then I was all ears. The two articles described an epidemic of chemical poisonings that had taken place in a newborn nursery. The window washer, James Merk, had been one of those kids. He'd been one of the subjects in both articles. Some of the other subjects had died. James had been more lucky. And his pediatrician had given him copies of the articles. They were his only claim to fame. And he didn't have very much else going for him.

"High school dropout?" I said.

"Yep," Vic replied.

"Negligence?" I asked.

"No question about it."

"So the question you're asking me is causation?" Had the toxic exposure that had been so thoroughly documented in the medical literature caused brain injury resulting in his becoming a high school dropout?

"You got it."

"Send him up to see me, and send me all his records."

"They're already in the mail."

"And the articles."

"Of course."

Evaluating a patient referred by a lawyer in order to render an "expert opinion" is not very different from any other diagnostic evaluation; only the terms that are employed are a bit different. The patient who comes in for a neurological consultation wants to know the diagnosis and what that diagnosis means to his or her life, that is, the prognosis, and may or may not ask, in passing, what causes whatever particular disease has just been diagnosed.

Diagnosis.

Prognosis.

Etiology.

The lawyer who refers a plaintiff for neurological evaluation wants to know the same things, but in different terms.

Damages. What has been injured? What functions or abilities has the patient lost?

Permanency. Is the damage permanent?

Causation. Did the incident cause the damage?

All more probably than not, to a reasonable degree of medical certainty.

The package reached my office long before James Merk did. That gave me the opportunity to read all about him in preparation for his examination. There was no history of neurological impairment such as walking difficulty, visual loss, and so on. In all probability, his damages, if any, would be some degree of intellectual impairment. In order to blame any one cause for that, there had to be evidence that no other sufficient cause for such injuries was documented in the medical records.

None was. His parents and siblings were all of average intelligence. He had been the only one of the four children in the family to have school problems. All told, there was no evidence of a hereditary cause of retardation. His mother's pregnancy had been totally uneventful. She had no illnesses of any sort. She'd taken no drugs. She didn't drink. The delivery had been a breeze. These negatives were not absolute proof. Not in a scientific sense. In medicine, you have to live with the fact that absence of proof is not proof of absence. But this was a question of civil law. The test was "more probably than not." A negative history was more than sufficient for these purposes.

On to the medical literature. I read all that there was to read about the epidemic of "hot" phenol poisoning that had affected infant-boy Merk, before he had even been given his full name. Had it occurred in another age, it would have been called a plague, but today we use the term *epidemic,* for that's just what it was, an epidemic — the sudden occurrence of a disease that wasn't supposed to occur.

The epidemic first came to light in April of 1967. A peculiar new syndrome burst out, involving a number of newborn children in the nursery of a small hospital in St. Louis. The hospital was an obstetric facility that had a total of twenty-six beds and a similar number of bassinets in the newborn nursery. None of the doctors had ever seen anything quite like it before. At first the babies were entirely normal; then, without any warning, their clothing and brows became drenched with sweat, but the children continued to nurse avidly. In less than a day, they started to have temperatures with fevers up to 103°F. Their respiratory rates increased and their breathing became labored. As far as the doctors could tell by listening, their chests were entirely clear. Other common findings included rapid heartbeats, enlarged livers, and irritability. This was soon followed by severe lethargy and decreased responsiveness. Loss of appetite, vomiting, and diarrhea, the common accompaniments of infection in the neonatal period, were notably not there. Stiffness of the neck and convulsions, the classic signs of meningitis or brain fever, were also absent. Skin rashes or other evidence of inflammation or irritation of the skin were not seen.

Laboratory tests frequently showed a change in acid-base balance, some protein in the urine, and some increase in the blood urea nitrogen. A "pneumonia" or "bronchiolitis" was seen on chest X rays. Bacterial and viral cultures of blood, cerebrospinal fluid, urine, nose, throat, and stool all showed nothing. Two of the children died, and postmortem studies of these cases revealed very little. Not enough to make any diagnosis at all.

When it started, the sweating syndrome struck four of the twenty-five infants in the nursery. The first of the four, tentatively diagnosed as having an infection, died on April 17, after treatment with antibiotics. The possibility of a toxic cause occurred to one of the residents who was assigned to the newborn nursery. On April 18, two infants with the sweating syndrome were transferred to a larger hospital in St. Louis, and because nothing else had helped previous patients, they were both given exchange transfusions. In this process, the child's blood is slowly removed and replaced by fresh donor's blood. This procedure is designed to help remove any foreign or toxic substance that might be in the baby's blood. Both children dramatically improved. On April 23, another infant, who had had a fever since April 18, was recognized as having the same syndrome and treated in the same way and recovered.

The St. Louis Health Department ordered the nursery closed on April 24. After a thorough cleaning, it reopened May 3. However, in the following two weeks, four more infants became ill. Among them was yet another fatal case. The disease in this infant progressed so rapidly that there was no chance to transfer the baby and perform an exchange transfusion. The nursery was closed for a second time, and the Health Department increased its efforts to find the cause of the sickness.

With most of his key people tied up in the case, Dr. Earl Smith, the St. Louis Health Commissioner, sought additional help. He telephoned the Center for Disease Control (CDC) in Atlanta on May 29. That evening, two members of the Center's epidemiology group arrived in St. Louis. By the time of their arrival on the scene, the focus of the search had shifted entirely away from possible bacteria and viruses to chemicals that might have gotten into the nursery and hospital. It had been the exchange transfusions, designed to remove toxins in the blood, that had saved many of the babies, not the antibiotics. A number of items were checked, including a solid-stick evaporating deodorizer that had been used in the nursery continuously for four years, an insecticide spray that had been used monthly in the hospital (but not in the nursery) for two years, drugs and baby formulas, and a disinfectant used on surfaces in contact with the infants. The laundry was also checked.

An important clue was discovered by a Dr. L. E. Loveless, a consulting chemist for the city's health department. Examining blood from the first eight patients via thin-layer chromatography, Dr. Loveless discovered that all the infants had some unknown phenolic chemical in their bodies. However, he could not identify exactly what phenol was present. The disinfectant was implicated immediately, since it was a mixture of several phenols, including hexachlorophene, one of the active ingredients of Dial soap. The investigators noted that the hospital had a "dedicated" cleaning woman, who used this disinfectant quite liberally around the nursery.

The parts of the picture implicating the disinfectant seemed to fit well. Dr. Alexander Langmuir, chief of CDC's epidemiology program, originally thought that the cause involved absorption of this germ-killing phenol through the skin, and the CDC was prepared to recommend that all hospitals use such phenolic compounds with extreme care. However, Dr. Smith and his chemists were not sure the evidence was clear-cut enough for such a recommendation.

The nursery was cleaned again. The original hexachlorophene-containing germicide was replaced, and all equipment previously treated with it was either discarded or freed of all phenolic residues by extensive cleaning with alcohol. New linens and diapers were purchased. The nursery reopened July 11.

And all went well, for more than a month. But on August 29, an eight-day-old infant broke out with severe sweating. Again, an exchange transfusion was performed and the infant rapidly recovered. And once again, the nursery was closed. A review of the records of all newborns revealed that six infants had had a mild form of the syndrome during July and August, but only after they had gone home from the nursery.

Hexachlorophene was not the cause. It had been eliminated and children continued to get ill. The cause had to be something else. But what? The investigators were baffled. It appeared that every source of phenols had been checked and double-checked. No other source had been found, but some sort of phenol had been in the infants' blood. What phenol? From where? In early September, Dr. Robert W. Armstrong, a CDC epidemiology officer who had just arrived in St. Louis, found the key to the puzzle. In the basement of the hospital, in a closet at the side of the laundry area, he came upon two 100-pound cardboard drums, each half the size of a common oil drum. One was virtually empty. The other, although opened, was almost entirely full. That one had just recently been delivered to the hospital. Obviously, this product was still in use.

Dr. Armstrong had been looking for any chemical that might be absorbed through the skin. The two large drums were turned so that their labels faced the wall. Armstrong turned them around. The labels identified the contents as an antimicrobial laundry neutralizer and brightener "for control of mildew and odor-causing bacteria." The active ingredients included pentachlorophenol as well as other phenol derivatives containing chlorine.

Armstrong had found what CDC was later to call "a previously overlooked source of phenols." Even though one of the drums had been in the hospital since March 1966, and even though the search for a source of phenols had been intensive, no one at the hospital was aware of the detergent's ingredients. The investigators now had a new and convincing picture of the cause of the sweating disease. In looking back, it became obvious that the symptoms of the sweating syndrome were very similar to the symptoms that had been described in the few known cases of industrial accidental poisonings resulting from overexposure to pentachlorophenol.

Thin-layer chromatography of the serum and urine of the child who had become ill on August 29 revealed a phenolic derivative with characteristics identical to those detected in the previous cases. Further chemical studies proved that the abnormal chemical in the urine and serum of the August 29 patient was pentachlorophenol. Hexachlorophene was entirely off the hook. Pentachlorophenol was also found in freshly laundered diapers from the nursery.

The label that Dr. Armstrong had seen when he turned the drums around also carried a critical warning: "Must not be used for laundering diapers or hospital linens." The warning was one of several, the most prominent being: "Keep out of reach of children. Harmful if swallowed! Causes skin irritation!"

Other investigators from the CDC proved that an identical epidemic had occurred in Cavalier, North Dakota, in 1966. This had involved a dozen or so newborns who had been exposed to the same detergent and had developed the same sweating syndrome. As a result of these incidents, the CDC published a warning that "pediatricians, hospital administrators, housekeepers, and local health authorities should check commercial diaper services and hospital laundries to ensure that this product is not in use."

As soon as I finished my review of the literature, I called Vic. Much of his case was already in place. Negligence, he felt, was easy to prove. Here was a product that warned against its use for laundering diapers or any hospital linens but, despite this, had been sold to an obstetric facility. Not a general hospital with an obstetrical service, but an obstetrical hospital, per se. What else were they going to use it for? That was obviously a no-no. He had filed suit against both the manufacturer and the hospital. The former shouldn't have sold it, and the latter shouldn't have bought it or used it. The warning was there on the cans for everyone to see. The next step was up to me.

I examined James Merk in my office. His general neurological exam was normal. At my request, one of our neuropsychologists also evaluated him. His findings weren't as benign. As expected, James had evidence of altered brain function. The combination of a normal overall examination and abnormal intelligence suggested a mild-to-moderate widespread insult to both hemispheres of his brain — just what one would see as residual damage from a toxic brain insult ("a toxic encephalopathy"). More importantly, my exam, as well as that of the neuropsychologist, had failed to un-cover any evidence suggesting any other possible etiology.

I gave my deposition about six months later. The lawyer who took it represented the manufacturer. The whole process lasted less than an hour and a half. He went over my CV very briefly, then my list of publications, how I spent my time, and got on to my opinions in the case of James Merk.

"Why were you retained in this case as you understand your job?"

"Well, my job was to give opinions to the best of my medical judgment whether or not any alteration in brain function, any deviation from normal in the function of the brain of James Merk, more likely than not could have been related to his documented toxic exposure."

"Well, Doctor, based on your review of the medical records furnished to you, your review of the literature on pentachlorophe-nol, your diagnosis, and your review of the psychologist's report, what opinions have you formed in this case concerning the effect, if any, of pentachlorophenol on James Merk?"

"Well, I have two opinions. One is that Mr. Merk did have a toxic encephalopathy as a newborn, caused by pentachlorophenol;

the second is that he now has a borderline level of intellectual function and that the most likely cause of this is the toxic encephalopathy that took place during the newborn period."

"All right. Doctor, what specifically do you base those opinions on?"

"Well, they're based on two different sets of reasoning. One is that he did have toxic exposure. This is well documented in the medical literature. He's included as one of the patients who had toxic exposure in the published studies. The children with this toxic exposure had irritability and lethargy and were thought by their own physicians to be so seriously ill neurologically that they frequently had spinal taps. Spinal taps are performed only when the physician believes that the patient has evidence of neurologic disease.

"So James had a disease which included, during its acute phase, central nervous system dysfunction. And now he has evidence of brain injury. The second line of reasoning is that I could find no other adequate explanation that could have been the cause of this."

That was it.

At the trial, things did not go quite so easily. I gave the same opinion, but this time I was cross-examined by a different lawyer, an older, more experienced trial lawyer, who attacked my opinions.

"Doctor, are you aware of any published authority that concludes that pentachlorophenol and exposure thereto adversely affects the central nervous system in humans?"

"I actually know of no published data on this question. I know of no follow-up studies on exposed individuals. Only such a study could definitively refute or support that conclusion."

"Would you agree with the statement that pentachlorophenol has never caused an effect on the central nervous system?"

"Absolutely not. The exposed infants were irritable and then became lethargic. Those are neurological symptoms due to problems within the central nervous system. That does not support any notion that pentachlorophenol does not affect the brain. Just the opposite."

"What are you basing that on, Doctor?"

"The exposed kids were sick. They had an encephalopathy when they were exposed to it. That is an effect on the nervous system. On the brain. Brain dysfunction. Pure and simple."

"What clinical findings or actual data can you cite, if any, to support that?"

"They were irritable and lethargic. If you would like to supply me with another cause for their changes in behavior, I'll accept it. I can't find one. They went into coma. I always thought loss of consciousness was evidence of central nervous system dysfunction. Perhaps you know another cause. I don't."

"Doctor, are you aware of any studies at all that show a different effect of pentachlorophenol on the brain?"

"In man?"

"Yes."

"I'm not aware of any studies that ever even attempted to look at that issue."

"So, you're not aware of any studies that were ever done that support your conclusion?"

"I'm not aware of any studies, period."

"Doctor, is it your opinion that pentachlorophenol causes brain injury?"

"It is my opinion that in this instance the toxic encephalopathy that occurred in this young lad more probably than not is the cause of any present brain abnormality that he has."

"Okay. It is accurate, though, is it not, Doctor, that the medical literature that you've read does not show any causative relationship between pentachlorophenol poisoning and any permanent brain injury, is that correct?"

"No. It is not. What is accurate to say is that the medical reports are silent on this issue. The children who did not die recovered. Whether their learning was normal or not is not addressed in those articles. They are silent on that question. No one ever looked."

He suddenly switched gears. It was a familiar tactic. If you can't attack a man's opinions, attack the man.

"You claim to spend half of your time treating patients."

"Yes, sir."

"Let's look at your CV. At the section called presentations. Now those are all papers you presented at various meetings?"

"Yes, sir. I or one of the other coauthors."

"Well, let's look at 1973, shall we?"

We did.

He then, without bothering to give any dates, listed all the international meetings at which I had had presentations in the next six years.

Barcelona.

Rome.

Paris.

Vienna.

Jerusalem.

Montreal.

London, five different times.

The implication was clear. He had mentioned one year and twelve meetings. How could I treat patients as I wandered endlessly around the globe?

"So you went to all these meetings?"

"No."

"But you said you did!"

"No. I said I or one of my coauthors did. I never went to half of those meetings. I may go to one a year."

"Rome. Did you go there?"

"No."

"Montreal?"

"No."

"London?"

"Yes."

"How often?"

"Four or five times."

"So you think nothing of just whipping off to London. It's just like a simple trip to St. Louis?" he added sarcastically.

"Just about," I agreed. "Unless it rains."

"What's rain got to do with it?"

"If it rains, it takes longer to drive to St. Louis than it does to fly to London."

That night the case was settled. The attorney had not been able to attack either my opinion or me successfully. He was no longer willing to leave it up to a jury. Instead, he made an offer that Vic was willing to accept. The lawyer had broached what to me was the most interesting question. The sweating syndrome had been a medical detective story of the first order. A new disease. A local epidemic. A plague. Like Legionnaire's disease. And the cause had been found. End of story. But was it? The victims in this story were not adults. They were newborn children. Most of them survived, but were the survivors normal? That was impossible to tell. Mild degrees of brain dysfunction cannot be detected until the children are much older. But the kids got better, went home, and once steps were taken to prevent any new outbreaks, once the disease was prevented, the true mission of the CDC, the story ended. But it wasn't over. Not for James Merk. For him, it will never be over. He still carries his article with him wherever he goes.

AUTHOR'S NOTE

The most important articles about James Merk and his acute disease are:

1. A. M. Robson, et al., "Pentachlorophenol Poisoning in a Nursery for Newborn Infants. I. Clinical Features and Treatment." *Journal of Pediatrics* 75: 309–316, 1969.
2. R. W. Armstrong, et al., "Pentachlorophenol Poisoning in a Nursery for Newborn Infants. II. Epidemiologic and Toxicologic Studies." *Journal of Pediatrics* 75: 317–325, 1969.

As far as I know, the exact fate of the other surviving children remains unknown. No one has systematically sought them out, which is not surprising. They all had different physicians and they scattered to different places. All they had in common was being poisoned by the same product in the same hospital. It is unlikely that either the manufacturer or the hospital ever wanted to find out exactly how well they did.

As I was completing this reminiscence, I recalled another, similar, story from the 1950s. A manufacturer of baby formula changed the production process in one of its plants. Shortly thereafter, an epidemic of severe seizures erupted, involving scores of young infants. No one knew what the cause of these seizures was. They were different from other seizures. Anticonvulsants didn't stop the seizures, but putting the children into the hospital did — almost any hospital.

The epidemiologists had a field day. They found the common thread. All the children used the same formula. The new process, it appears, destroyed vitamin B-6, and the children suffered from acute loss of B-6, resulting in seizures, seizures that could be stopped only by giving them B-6. This was why hospitalization stopped the seizures. In the 1950s, hospitals still made their own formulas, and B-6 was present in all such hospital-made formulas.

End of story.

Or was it? Vitamin deficiency can cause brain damage. So can recurrent seizures. Did these kids grow up to have normal brains? We don't know. Why? Because no one ever looked.

The last time I saw Vic, I asked him how James was doing.

"Fine," he said. "He's still washing windows and showing everyone and anyone his articles."

"I guess Andy Warhol was right," I said.

"Who?"

There may be some advantages to living in southern Illinois.

CHAPTER EIGHT

Therapeutic Misadventure

Some consulting rooms are full of complainers . . .
professionals for whom pain is a career.

> — Francis Dudley-Hart, M.D.,
> *to the British Medical Association.*
> *Quoted in the London* DailyTelegraph,
> *July 17, 1974.*

Mrs. Lillian Schwartz was not a well woman. At least not if you listened to her. She was seventy years old and she hadn't felt good in years. Dozens of years. And the doctors never seemed to do anything that really helped. If it wasn't one thing, it was another. Her heart was fine. Chest pain was one pain she didn't have. Thank God. Every year her EKG was normal. And no headaches. She had never had headaches. Her late husband, Milton, he had had headaches. Regular migraines. Every week. So she knew all about headaches. And high blood pressure. Milton had had that, too. And a fatal heart attack ten years ago. She still lived by herself. Who needed another husband to bury? And she wasn't going to be a burden on her two daughters. They already had enough problems. More than enough.

So did she. But she managed despite all her aches and pains. She cleaned her house. She went to the store. She even dragged herself to see her doctor. Dr. Benjamin Parks. Once a week she went to see him. She had arthritis. Everywhere — her hands, her knees, her back. Especially in her back.

Dr. Parks listened to her and changed her medicine. Aspirin. Motrin. Butazolidin. Nuprin.

Her back kept right on hurting. And it got harder and harder for her to drag herself around.

So finally he said she should go to the hospital. She went. To St. Michael's Hospital. But she didn't get any better.

Nothing seemed to help. Not bed rest. Not traction. Not the injection of cortisone. Not the pain killers. Not physical therapy. Not the muscle relaxants.

Dr. Parks asked a neurosurgeon to see her in consultation. A Doctor Keith Cooper. A nice, refined, polite man. Dr. Cooper told her that she might need an operation.

For what?

Spinal stenosis.

What was that?

Arthritis of her back pushing in on the nerves.

Was that what was causing her pain?

He thought so.

Would the operation help the pain?

Yes.

Nothing else had helped. Was he certain the operation would?

Yes.

She was ready for it.

First, they had to do a test.

What test?

A myelogram.

What was that?

He explained it to her. A little discomfort. Maybe some pain. But a safe test.

When would he do it?

First, he would talk to Dr. Parks, then he would schedule it, probably in the next day or two.

That was fine with her.

Cooper talked to Parks and told him what he thought and what he wanted to do.

That was okay with Dr. Parks. If Mrs. Schwartz needed an operation, she would become Dr. Cooper's problem. She could see him weekly for the next couple of years. He had put in his time.

Later that night, Parks went through a number of the throwaway journals that he got each week merely by being a physician: *Medical Economics, Postgraduate Medicine.* And several others. For no particular reason he suddenly recalled an article he had read a couple of years earlier about using colchicine for patients with long-standing back pain that hadn't responded to other forms of treatment. Colchicine was a powerful drug, one of the mainstays in the treatment of gout. It was usually given orally. On rare occasions, in acute gout, it is given intravenously. It works faster that way.

Parks had treated lots of patients with colchicine. They had all had gout. He had usually given it orally, but he had used it intravenously more than just a couple of times. He had never given it to Lillian Schwartz. It was one of the few things he had never tried. It might be worth a try. Why not? Anything was better than major back surgery. And safer.

Of course, she didn't have gout, but colchicine worked in other forms of arthritic disease. In back disease. He could remember the article. It had been in one of those throwaway journals he had thrown away.

Colchicine it would be.

Parks called the hospital and talked to the intern, a Dr. Ahmed Hassan. Dr. Parks told Dr. Hassan that he wanted Mrs. Schwartz to get two milligrams of colchicine.

"Orally?"

"No. I want it to work faster than that."

"Intravenously?"

Parks thought for a moment. "No. Make it intrathecally. That's where her problem is. In the spinal fluid space around her spinal cord and nerves."

"Intrathecally," Dr. Hassan repeated. Dr. Hassan hoped that he didn't have to do the spinal tap himself in order to put the colchicine into the intrathecal space surrounding the spinal cord. Before he got a chance to ask, Dr. Parks relieved his worries.

"Dr. Cooper is doing a myelogram tomorrow morning. Have the pharmacy send up the colchicine, send it to X ray with her, and Cooper can give it after he's done the myelogram. He has to do a spinal tap for the myelogram. There's no reason to do two of them."

"No reason at all," Dr. Hassan agreed.

So the intern wrote the order as instructed:

> Colchicine 2 mg. intrathecally.
> To be given at time of myelogram.
> Colchicine to radiology with patient.

Dr. Hassan had never heard of anyone giving colchicine intrathecally. He had never read about it in any of his textbooks. But that didn't surprise him. That was why he had come to the U.S. for an internship and a residency. Afterward he would go back to Iraq — maybe.

The nurse transcribed the orders just the way they were written. She had never seen an order for intrathecal colchicine. She didn't stop to look it up. She didn't ask any other nurse. She didn't question the doctor. She just transcribed the order and sent the requisition to the pharmacy.

The pharmacist filled the order as written. He had never seen an order for intrathecal colchicine. He had never even heard of using colchicine intrathecally. He didn't stop to look it up. He didn't ask any of the other pharmacists about it. He just took a two-milligram vial of colchicine and sent it off to the nursing station.

There the nurse took the colchicine and taped it to Mrs. Schwartz's chart. This was not the same nurse who had made out the requisition. The nurse also had never heard of using colchicine intrathecally. But all she did was tape the medicine to the chart so it would get to radiology when Mrs. Schwartz did.

Mrs. Schwartz was rolled off to radiology with her chart and the vial containing two milligrams of colchicine.

Dr. Cooper was there waiting for her.

He looked at the chart and wondered about the vial of medicine. He knew what colchicine was. It was for gout.

But an intrathecal injection?

He had never heard of that.

That's because he was a neurosurgeon. He didn't treat gout. That was something that internists treated. Internists like Parks.

Cooper did the spinal tap.

He put in the dye for the myelogram.

The radiology technician took the films. Cooper looked at them. Not enough spinal stenosis to warrant surgery. No operation for

Mrs. Schwartz. Then he remembered the vial, drew the colchicine into a syringe, and injected it. Intrathecally.

That night, Mrs. Schwartz thought that her feet felt numb.

And the next morning she had trouble moving her toes. Her feet seemed to drag more than usual when she went to the bathroom.

By lunchtime, her legs were numb.

By dinner she couldn't move her legs.

Dr. Parks had no idea what was wrong. A reaction to the myelogram dye, he suggested.

Or an infection.

He decided to give her some steroids.

The next morning her arms were paralyzed and she felt short of breath. By lunchtime, she had lapsed into a coma.

The daughters were beside themselves. What had happened to their mother?

Parks wasn't sure.

Neither was Cooper.

Or the neurologist they called in, a Dr. Boyer.

Each one told the daughters the same story. They had no idea what had happened. It was probably an allergic reaction to the dye. They would do all they could to maintain her respiration and blood pressure and she might recover.

"Fully?" the family asked.

"Completely?" they inquired.

Why not?

The chart told a different story.

Parks was certain that she had diffuse toxicity of the brain and spinal cord from colchicine. So was Boyer. And even Dr. Cooper. And all of the other doctors involved in her care. And she had no chance of recovery. Within a week, she was brain-dead. The EEGs showed absolutely no brain activity at all.

But her heart went on and on.

And the doctors kept scratching their heads in front of the daughters and telling them that there was still a chance that their mother might recover.

Fully?

Why not?

Mrs. Schwartz's brother was a doctor. He was retired and living in Florida. He had been talking to the daughters. He had never heard of such an allergic reaction.

After a week without any improvement, one daughter asked Dr. Parks to call their uncle. Parks did nothing.

Two weeks went by. Uncle Irving had not been called. The daughters asked Parks to send their uncle a copy of the records. Parks did nothing.

Four weeks. Mrs. Schwartz remained on the respirator, in a coma. Could she still recover?

Yes.

Fully?

Why not?

Did anyone know what had happened?

No.

The daughter sent a letter to Dr. Parks, formally requesting that all records be sent to their uncle, Dr. Irving Katzman. He had very little choice. He wrote a letter to the Illinois State Medical Insurance Corporation, which carried his malpractice insurance. He felt he had to notify them what had happened and, in so doing, cover his own backside. He told them that a patient of his had inadvertently been given colchicine, by an intrathecal manner. "There was," he wrote, "a communication problem between the neurosurgeon and myself and a resident. I suggested that the medication be given intravenously. This was misinterpreted and an order was written to give it intrathecally at the time of a myelogram. I had personally had no experience with intrathecal colchicine and, as far as I know, it has not been given before in this method." He went on to suggest that the effects of colchicine on the central nervous system could be quite severe. His patient had developed a severe neurological problem following her myelogram, and "although there were multiple reasons why this could have occurred, the colchicine given in that manner could be a reasonable cause of her problem." The patient was still alive. She was still under his care. There was no medical suit pending, as far as he knew. He had "informed the family that the entire syndrome could be due to dye injected for a myelogram."

Six weeks. Irving Katzman had still received nothing. The daughters sent Parks another letter. He wrote a letter to Dr. Katzman. In it he enclosed the "pertinent laboratory results regarding Lillian Schwartz." He briefly relayed her history: she had had pain in her low back, which had been increasing for some time. The pain traveled into both lower extremities, and there was also pain on flexion of neck. He told Katzman that his sister had had a long-standing history of unremitting low-back pain and intolerance of almost every analgesic or anti-inflammatory drug used. He suggested hospitalization to her; she agreed, and was admitted. Following admission, there was a consultation with Dr. Cooper, a neurosurgeon. He suggested a myelogram. The myelogram showed multiple levels of modest involvement but no clear indication for surgery. "Hours after the myelogram, her pain worsened and she developed a severe neurological problem." Whether it was inflammatory or toxic, he was "not sure."

He ended his note with an equally noncommittal summary. "She is currently in a coma and all steps are being taken to give her total support with hope for eventual recovery. Enclosed are the lab slips and old CAT scan. Cordially yours."

Eight weeks after the myelogram, Ms. Schwartz was still no better. In a few days her Medicare benefits would be exhausted. Two days later, she developed pneumonia, which no one treated, and she died.

The family requested an autopsy to find out what had happened. The pathologist at St. Michael's hated doing autopsies. He read the record. As he saw it, there was an unexplained death following an invasive procedure. That made it a case for the coroner. The coroner's office did the autopsy. They discovered that Mrs. Schwartz's brain and spinal cord had turned into pea soup.

The coroner's final diagnosis was simple and direct. Diffuse necrosis of the brain due to colchicine toxicity caused by a therapeutic misadventure.

In due time, the family lawyer asked for copies of the death certificate to close Mrs. Schwartz's bank accounts and to take care of some other legal matters. He took the time to read it. Diffuse necrosis of the brain due to colchicine toxicity caused by therapeutic misadventure.

Misadventure, hell. The doctors had killed Mrs. Schwartz. He told the family and referred them to another lawyer, Jim Gould.

He specialized in malpractice. Gould asked me to review the case.

I did. I read all the records and then we discussed the case over the phone.

Causation was obvious.

The colchicine had killed her. As far as I knew, no one had ever used colchicine intrathecally before. Medicines are rarely given that way. Intrathecal administration puts the medicine inside the blood-brain barrier. That barrier is designed to protect the brain from toxins. Giving it that way was crazy.

But who was at fault?

Parks. According to the record, he had ordered the intrathecal colchicine.

But he had apparently changed his story. He claimed that he had ordered it to be given intravenously, not intrathecally. The intern had misunderstood. It was the intern's fault. It was the old story of poor little John Dean leading Richard Nixon astray. Ollie North setting White House policy. People will believe anything.

The intern? Dr. Hassan was certain he'd understood exactly what Dr. Parks had ordered. It was a strange order, but he was just an intern. How could he challenge the doctor's order? He, too, was at fault.

The nurses? They had just followed orders. Like good little nurse. In reality, they had an obligation to check on any peculiar use of a medication.

The pharmacist? He, too, had followed orders. The doctors wanted colchicine to give intrathecally. They got it.

Had he ever heard of that before? No.

But he was paid to monitor drugs. And drug safety. That's why pharmacists go to pharmacy school for five years or more and become licensed. Not just to learn to count to twenty-four.

The neurosurgeon? In my mind, he was the real culprit. He was supposed to be the expert on the nervous system. He knew how vulnerable the brain is. He knew about the role of the blood-brain barrier in protecting the brain. And he gave the injection.

He claimed that he was merely a technician. He was doing a myelogram. Parks ordered the colchicine. He gave it. Like any other technician, he had merely been following orders.

"No one had followed orders that well since the days of the Third Reich," I mumbled.

As far as I was concerned, everyone shared in the responsibility. Gould should sue them all.

A few weeks later, Gould took Parks's deposition. Each defendant in any suit involving numerous defendants has one of two choices. The defendant can claim that neither he nor anyone did anything wrong, or that one of the other defendants screwed up. The concept that no one in this case did anything wrong would have been hard to swallow.

Gould, of course, asked the questions. It took only ten minutes for him to get down to the issues.

"Is it fair to say, Doctor," Gould inquired, "that a paper you had read prompted you to use the colchicine for the relief of disc pain in Mrs. Schwartz?"

"It was that paper, and the references to the paper," Parks replied.

"Did that paper advocate a particular route of administration?"

"It mentioned IV use."

"Did the author mention any other use?"

"Oral use."

"Anything else?"

"That's all that I remember."

"So, the only method by which colchicine was used, as you understood it, in terms of route of administration, was IV or oral, is that right?"

"Yes, sir."

"Had you seen anything anywhere in the literature, anywhere in the history of medicine that ever advocated the intrathecal administration of the drug?" Gould asked.

"Never," Parks admitted.

Parks was going to stick to the story he had written to his insurance company. It wasn't his fault. It wasn't his order they were following. A misunderstanding. A communication problem. Their fault, not his.

"Had you ever used the drug in an intrathecal manner?"

"Never."

"Are you familiar, Doctor, with the pharmacology of colchicine?"

"In reference to joint disease."

"Doctor, are you aware of colchicine being used intramuscularly or subcutaneously?"

"I have never used it that way."

"Can you think of any reason why one would not administer colchicine IM?"

"I think it is a very irritating chemical."

"And, what would you expect to happen if it was administered IM?"

"Cellular death."

"And, what would one expect to happen if it was administered subcutaneously?"

"Soft-tissue death and irritation."

"What is it about the drug that leads you to conclude that it would be irritating and would result in cell death if administered IM or subcutaneously?"

"Because of its ability to be picked up by cells, and its ability to cause death of these cells very rapidly."

"Now, in terms of its IV administration, for what — what precaution, if you — strike that. How do you administer it IV?"

"The way I have always used it intravenously is that I first get into the vein, and then, when I inject it, I make sure that we have a rapidly flowing intravenous site, and I usually wash the material through locally. I use dextrose in water, or intravenous saline after the colchicine is administered, and I make sure that the colchicine is directly in the vein and doesn't slip into the subcutaneous tissues, because where this has happened, I have seen intense pain caused to patients."

And now it was established that Parks knew that colchicine was a dangerous drug, a drug that was capable of rapidly killing cells.

"When did you first see the order on Mrs. Schwartz's chart for intrathecal colchicine?"

"It had to be the next day, the day after the myelogram."

"Did you assume that the colchicine had been injected pursuant to that order?"

"I assumed it had been."

"And what did that mean to you?"

"It meant," he began and then stopped and started over hesitantly. "I had no experience with this, I did not know what it meant. I knew this was a totally unorthodox method of the administration of colchicine."

"Based upon your experience and knowledge of colchicine as a drug, what did you think about its potential effect, or potential for irritation, having been injected intrathecally?"

"I think my notes in the hospital records clearly stated that the patient had an irritation to the central nervous system from the drug," he replied firmly.

Those were, of course, his notes on the record he had failed to send to Dr. Katzman.

"So you knew it was an irritant?"

"Yes, I did."

"And you knew that it would cause irritation to the central nervous system, correct?"

"Yes."

"And you knew it never before in the history of mankind had ever been injected that way?"

"That's right."

"Now, having known those things, was there anything that you could have done at that time to reverse the potential effect of that colchicine instillation into the spinal canal?"

"I honestly believe by the time I had noted these things there was nothing I could do, because of the very rapid uptake of the drug from the spinal fluid, and it probably was inside the cells long before the patient developed symptoms, and before I returned to the hospital to see her the next day. So, I did not feel that there was anything, when I saw her, that I could do to reverse this, or I certainly would have done so."

"So that by the day after the myelogram, it was all over?"

"I think it was. There was nothing that could be done at that point."

Gould went back to the order of the colchicine. Parks stated that he had not ordered it to be given intrathecally. No one was going to pin this one on him. He was going to pin it on someone else. That lousy Arab intern.

So it had been Dr. Hassan's mistake.

Yes. He must have misunderstood.

It was entirely his fault.

Entirely?

"One hundred percent."

Gould then talked about the order itself. Was the order itself sent to the pharmacy?

"Yes."

"So that anybody in pharmacy who got a copy of that order would not only know the drug requested, but the method of administration, is that right?"

"Yes. They get a copy of the exact order as it is written."

"And would it be fair to say that a pharmacist would know, upon looking at that order, that colchicine should not be injected intrathecally?"

"I am quite sure a pharmacist should know that," he admitted grudgingly. He could not maintain that the only guilty party was a single Arab intern. They were all to blame. They had killed his patient.

"And you would expect the nurse who sees the order and countersigns it to recognize that colchicine should not be injected intrathecally?"

"That's correct, sir," Parks answered promptly.

The attorneys for the other defendants were cringing. He had turned on them. They would not be a unified defense. There would be more mudslinging than in a presidential campaign. Well, they too could play that game. Hassan would swear he had not misunderstood the order. Not at all.

"And, would you have expected Dr. Hassan to recognize colchicine shouldn't be injected intrathecally?"

"That's correct."

"And you certainly would have expected Dr. Cooper to recognize this?"

"Yes, as well as myself."

"By the morning of the twentieth, then, there was absolutely no doubt in your mind that what occurred at the time of the myelogram shouldn't have occurred, is that correct?"

"I was quite sure that the route of administration was improper, and that this should not have been done."

"And that in terms of Lillian Schwartz's future, that was sealed before you saw her the next morning."

He nodded.

"You have to say your answer out loud so that the court reporter can transcribe it."

"Yes," he mumbled.

"Louder, please."

"Yes."

Gould sent me Parks's deposition. He also sent me copies of all the other depositions as they were taken. The other defendants pretty much said what was expected.

Hassan had followed orders. He had no doubt in his mind. Parks had said intrathecally. To send it along to radiology and have Dr. Cooper give it. He was only an intern. He'd never originated an order like that in his life. He didn't even know you could give medicine that way after a myelogram. Parks did. He gave the order.

Tit for tat.

The nurses had also merely followed orders.

And so had Cooper, the "technician."

But not the pharmacists. The hospital had ten pharmacists. Each of them denied ever having seen the order. Each of them denied ever having filled the order. It had been sent to the pharmacy. It had been seen. It had been filled.

By nobody at all.

It was time for my deposition.

Parks's lawyer, a man named Nelson, asked the first set of questions.

Did I have an opinion as to the cause of Mrs. Schwartz's neurological problem?

I did. Colchicine toxicity. "Due to," I added, "therapeutic misadventure."

Was I certain?

Absolutely. There was no other possible cause.

Had Dr. Parks deviated from the standard of care in the treatment he had rendered to Lillian Schwartz?

"Absolutely."

"Even if he ordered the colchicine to be given IV, as he testified, and not intrathecally?"

"Absolutely."

"How can you say that?"

"Easy. The only approved use for colchicine is gout. Mrs. Schwartz had arthritis and disc disease, not gout. There is no indication for colchicine in degenerative disc disease. None at all. I know of no competent authority that maintains there is."

"There is an entire body of authoritative literature on the use of intravenous colchicine in disc disease," he informed me.

"There is no such body of authoritative literature," I informed him.

"Do you deny that there are several articles by Dr. Karr in the medical literature?"

"There are no such articles in the medical literature."

Gould was beside himself. I was his only expert. I was impeaching myself. Nelson had the articles. I'd seen them. Gould had sent them to me.

"You deny the very existence of the articles by Dr. Karr?"

"I didn't say that. I denied and still deny that there is a single article in the recognized medical literature which advocates the use of IV colchicine for disc disease," I explained.

"Dr. Klawans has both impeached and contradicted himself," Nelson concluded. "I see no reason to hear his other opinions."

Gould was dying.

"I have done neither. Karr's articles exist. So do *Batman* comic books and *Hustler*. None of them represents competent medical authority. But they do exist."

"Karr's articles are part of the medical literature."

"They are not."

"They aren't?"

"No."

"Why not?"

"The medical literature is a body of printed material which has a recognized degree of authority. In journals, what constitutes that authority is fairly easy to define. The articles, once submitted to the journal, must be scrutinized and judged by appropriate authorities before being accepted for publication — a process called refereeing."

"And you're an expert on that."

"I do edit a medical journal," I said.

"Karr's articles were published in a medical journal."

"No. They were published in a nonrefereed, throw-away journal sent out by a drug company."

"So you arbitrarily decide what is and isn't a medical journal."

"Not me."

"Who?"

"The Library of Congress. They put together the index of all authoritative journals. It is called the *Index Medicus*. My journal is listed in the *Index Medicus*. The so-called journal in which Karr's article was published is not. I have a list of all the journals in the *Index Medicus* with me, if you'd like to see it. And the computer printout I got when I requested a list of all articles by Karr in the *Index Medicus*. There aren't any. None at all. None about colchicine for anything."

"I don't need to see those," Nelson replied.

"I do," Gould said, completely revived. I had more than rehabilitated myself. I had shown that Parks's use of colchicine in any manner for this patient had no support at all in the real medical literature. The paper he relied on did not exist. "Dr. Klawans has relied on those printouts. I want them marked as exhibits and attached to the record."

The reporter did just that. It was her job to follow orders.

The next two hours went by without incident. They got all of my opinions, one by one.

Intravenous colchicine was a deviation. The patient did not have gout.

Intrathecal colchicine was a deviation. It had killed Mrs. Schwartz.

Whoever ordered it had killed her. But everyone was at fault. The intern, Dr. Hassan, the nurses, the pharmacist, and Dr. Cooper.

There was also one other deviation. The failure of the physicians to tell the family the truth as to causation and prognosis was not acceptable. Lying was not within the standard of care.

Each of the defendants had his or her own lawyer. Each got to take a shot at me. They all followed the same scenario.

Didn't the nurse have the right to just follow the order?

No.

Or the pharmacist?

No.

Or the intern?

No.

Or the neurosurgeon?

Absolutely not.

"But he was merely acting as a technician, wasn't he?"

"No."

"He testified that he was."

"He lied."

"Dr. Klawans. That is a grave accusation."

"He sent Mrs. Schwartz a bill for the myelogram. A bill for fifteen hundred dollars. A bill which, in part, was paid by Medicare as a physician's professional fee. Not a technician's fee. You're right. Perhaps he didn't lie. But if he didn't lie, he defrauded Medicare. Personally, I don't think Cooper is a swindler. But I may be wrong. I've been wrong before."

It was getting late. They were now on the defensive. They had to do something to rehabilitate Cooper.

"Now, specifically with reference to this case, accepting for the moment Dr. Cooper's testimony, and you said you have read his deposition wherein he indicated that he was requested by Dr. Parks to administer the colchicine, at the completion of the myelogram, intrathecally, what, in your opinion, should Dr. Cooper have done before he administered that colchicine?"

"He should have known whether the intrathecal use of colchicine had been proved to be safe, and without that knowledge should have declined to do it."

"To your knowledge, as of December 1980, was colchicine being used experimentally for treatment of spinal arthritis by intrathecal injection?"

"Not that I am aware of."

"Are you aware of any literature, as of December of 1980, which would have advised Dr. Cooper that he should not have administered it in that fashion?"

"You mean a specific written admonition in the literature not to do that? Yes, there is. Well, to start with, the ampule is marked 'for intravenous use only.' The package insert also says it's approved only for intravenous use. And the entire literature on colchicine, which never once, as far as I am aware, mentioned that its safety within the spinal fluid space had ever been demonstrated."

"The information concerning the toxicity of colchicine and the effect it might have if administered intrathecally, are these the type of things that you would expect a neurosurgeon to know without researching as of December 1980?"

"Yes."

"In your opinion, wasn't Dr. Cooper justified in relying upon the representations of the internist, who is more familiar with the drug and uses it on a regular basis?"

"Absolutely not. He is in this matter the consultant on the neurological and neurosurgical aspect of that case and the expert thereupon. He must be the final arbiter of anything he puts into that space."

Did I know Dr. Cooper personally?

Not really.

He'd been in Chicago for many years. Was I aware of his excellent reputation as a neurosurgeon?

No.

Had I heard of him?

Yes.

But not of his excellent reputation?

He should have let it drop. "No."

Why not?

Because he didn't have one. He had lost privileges at at least one major hospital. That was why he had gone to St. Michael's Hospital. Everyone knew that.

Everyone?

As far as I knew, it was common knowledge.

My deposition was over.

I had made one error. Everyone did not know all about Dr. Cooper's problems. James Gould, for one, didn't. But now he did. And he pursued the issue tenaciously. If I knew and the medical community knew, shouldn't St. Michael's have known?

I thought they should have.

And done something about it?

Probably.

But did they know?

It took a couple of subpoenas and a couple of months, but he got the data. Cooper's surgical privileges had been permanently and irrevocably suspended at Chicago University Hospital, earlier in 1980. That fact, of course, had not been reported to the Illinois Department of Registration and Education.

Why not?

In Illinois, hospitals rarely, if ever, inform the state of such actions. And the state never seeks such information. Those doctors who lose their privileges at one hospital move to another. Cooper went to St. Michael's.

But did St. Michael's know any of this?

Yes. They had written to Chicago University Hospital about Cooper and had gotten an answer.

> In response to your letter of April 1, 1980, inquiring as to the circumstances under which Dr. Keith Cooper was the subject of action taken by this Hospital affecting his clinical privileges, the following is offered.
>
> In the spring of 1978 a Committee for the Study of Neurosurgical Indications and Complications was created to review all neurosurgical procedures performed in the Medical Center Hospitals during 1977. This Committee completed its work on September 1, 1978, and issued its report. On the basis of this report and the findings it contained, it was recommended to Dr. Cooper during the annual review of his privileges, which took place in late September 1978, that his privileges be modified. On September 25, 1978, Dr. Cooper filed an action against the Hospital seeking to enjoin any restriction of his privileges as suggested, but this complaint was voluntarily dismissed upon agreement of counsel for all par-

ties that Dr. Cooper would be provided a hearing on the issue of the modification of his privileges through the hearing mechanism existing under this Hospital's Medical Staff Bylaws, as well as a review conducted by physicians external to this Hospital. During this period Dr. Cooper also agreed to a modification of his privileges.

A review was conducted by three prominent external neurosurgeons on February 2 and 3, 1979, which essentially supported the findings of the Committee on the Study of Neurosurgical Indications and Complications. Thereafter, the hearing requested by Dr. Cooper was convened to determine if the clinical privileges of Dr. Cooper had been correctly restricted. During the pendency of these hearings, and, as a result of incidents involving the care and treatment of other patients by Dr. Cooper, all of Dr. Cooper's clinical privileges were summarily suspended on June 13, 1979.

On September 6, 1979, the committee reviewing the modification of Dr. Cooper's privileges issued its findings and held that the restriction of Dr. Cooper's privileges (as effected in September 1978) was reasonably based upon fact. As provided in the Bylaws, Dr. Cooper requested an appellate review of this finding, and upon completion of that review, the Hospital's Board of Directors on November 19, 1979, affirmed the modification of privileges.

Prior to this final board action on the modification of his privileges, Dr. Cooper on October 29, 1979, requested a hearing on the summary suspension of his privileges, which had been effected the previous June. A committee to conduct these hearings first met on November 21, 1979, and after several months of hearings reported on April 16, 1980, that the summary suspension of his clinical privileges was reasonably based upon fact. This finding was not appealed by Dr. Cooper.

Given the foregoing, the current status of Dr. Cooper's relationship with the Hospital is that he remains a member of the Medical Staff, but all of his clinical privileges have been indefinitely suspended.

I trust that the foregoing information is in sufficient detail

for you to understand the circumstances under which Dr.
Cooper's privileges were modified and suspended.

If you have any questions concerning the above information, please contact me.

St. Michael's knew and had done nothing. They needed neurosurgeons to keep the beds filled. They did not know the exact
details, of course.

Under Illinois law, hospitals may tell the state if they revoke or
limit a doctor's privileges. But hospitals are barred from disclosing
to anyone what the doctor actually did to prompt the action. That
information is "strictly confidential."

Each hospital decides on its own to whom it will grant staff
privileges. Only doctors with staff privileges are allowed to admit
and treat patients and perform surgery at that hospital.

St. Michael's had let Cooper in.

The case did not drag on much longer. There was never a trial. The
case was settled for somewhere between a half a million and a
million dollars. After all, the patient was seventy and enjoying ill
health.

But it did not end there.

St. Michael's took no action on the privileges of either Parks or
Cooper. That's the way the system works. But they hinted that
they might.

Cooper moved his practice to a suburban hospital.

His career was in reverse. He had to do something to change
that. But what? He decided to sue Chicago University Hospital.
They had treated him unfairly. He'd go to court and force them to
take him back. So he filed suit against Chicago. He pulled an Oscar
Wilde. And like Oscar Wilde, he, too, lost in the end.

The court found that there had been nothing wrong in what
Chicago University Hospital had done. Cooper had lost his privileges and now his entire reputation, justifiably.

But it did not end there.

The Chicago University Hospital viewed itself as "one of the
stops" on Dr. Cooper's sojourn through Chicago hospitals. A
sojourn marked by numerous malpractice suits. It was apparently

these suits that led to their reviewing, and then revoking, his surgical privileges.

But it did not end there.

With all the publicity of the court cases, the Department of Registration and Education had to do something.

They revoked Cooper's license.

He is now practicing neurosurgery in Saudi Arabia. Allah be praised.

Dr. Parks retired.

Dr. Hassan went on to take a residency in anesthesiology and never returned to Iraq. Would you?

The nurses and pharmacist are still following orders.

CHAPTER NINE

The Sleeping Killer

The feeling of sleepiness when you are not in bed and can't get
there is the meanest feeling in the world.

— E. W. Howe
Country Town Sayings

T ed Faber was a lawyer who specialized in tax law. He was also
a CPA, so tax law was second nature to him. His office was in
Chicago, but he had clients all over Illinois and the neighboring
states, and it wasn't unusual for him to travel to see his clients. It
was often easier and more efficient that way; there would never be
any question of the client not bringing along the right records. One
day in early April, just before the IRS deadline, Ted left Chicago
early in the morning and drove to Rock Island to see an old client.
They worked straight through the day and didn't finish up until
after eleven at night. They hadn't even stopped to eat but had
ordered some food to be delivered. Pizza. Not real Chicago pizza,
but what could one expect out in the sticks? Four hours later, as he
got into his car, Ted could still taste it.

What should he do? He had two choices. He could take a motel
room or drive home.

He was wiped out. He had worked now for four straight weeks
without taking a single day off. And he had worked at least twelve
to fourteen hours each day. He was only forty-seven but felt that
he was getting too old for this kind of schedule. Well, after four
more days, he could sleep for a week. He knew it would be easier
to check into some motel, but tomorrow was his daughter's birthday. She would be sixteen. Ted wanted to be home to give her her
present as soon as she woke up. It was a tradition that dated back
to her second birthday. He hadn't missed it once. And he sure as

hell wasn't going to miss this one. One more and there would be no more. She'd be off to college.

"Home, Jeeves," he said to himself. If he got too tired, he would pull off the road and take a nap in the car.

And that is just what he did. Less than halfway back to Chicago, he pulled off the road to sleep for a while. He knew it wasn't safe to go on without any sleep. It was just after one in the morning when he closed his eyes. In no time at all, he was asleep.

The next thing he knew, a cop was banging on the window. According to the clock on the dashboard, it was ten past three. He had slept for two hours.

The cop hit the window again.

Faber rolled the window down.

"Step out of the car," the policeman said gruffly. He was a state trooper.

"I was just taking a little nap, Officer," he began politely.

"Get out of the car," the trooper ordered.

It was obvious that the trooper meant business. Faber opened the door and got out.

The trooper grabbed him, threw him over the front hood, frisked him, pulled his arms behind him, and handcuffed him.

"What's that for?" Faber asked in surprise. "I was just taking a little nap."

"As if you didn't know, you bastard. One of the girls is dead. She was only sixteen years old. You killed her. Well, unfortunately for you, the other one is alive. She told us the whole story. It's too bad we don't have capital punishment for guys like you."

Ted Faber had no idea what the policeman was talking about. All he had done was stop on the roadside and take a little nap. That might have been a crime, but it didn't deserve this kind of treatment and certainly not capital punishment.

The girl who was still alive was another sixteen-year-old named Sherry Robertson. She had told the police the entire story. Sherry had been out with her friend Jodie Kerr. They had been at a party and stayed later than they should have, but not terribly late. They left at about one-thirty. They started to drive home but they ran out of gas. Jodie had been driving her brother's car. He never kept much gas in the car, and they just forgot to check. It had happened to them before. If only Jodie had remembered. Or if she had reminded her on the way to the party. If only . . .

The car stopped. They knew what was wrong, but they had no idea what to do. It was getting late; their parents would be really mad. They started to walk down the road, but no cars came by. Finally, they got to the highway and saw a parked car.

And someone was in the car.

They walked up to the car quietly.

It was a man. He was alone. He was sleeping.

Jodie knocked on the window. Lightly at first. Then harder. And harder.

The man suddenly sat up straight and looked out the window at them.

All he did was look.

He didn't roll down the window.

He just looked. Stared. With a strange look in his eyes. As if he were drunk.

Or afraid.

Then he started the car and pulled away.

"You SOB," Jodie yelled after him. "You bastard."

He must have heard her curses, because the next thing Sherry saw was the car slowing down and then turning around to face toward them.

"He's coming back," Jodie said. "We'll get a ride."

All of a sudden the car speeded up. Sherry could hear the squealing of the tires. It was headed straight for them.

The lights almost blinded her.

Sherry froze in place.

Like a jackrabbit.

Then she jumped to the right and screamed.

Jodie did neither.

The car hit her with a sickening thud.

Jodie flew into the air.

Still she never screamed. Not once. She landed halfway across the highway. The car was heading off toward Chicago, like a bat out of hell.

Sherry ran over to Jodie. Jodie was moaning softly. Thank God, she was still alive. "That fucking SOB!"

Suddenly Sherry knew that it wasn't over. She looked down the road. The car was coming back again.

Faster than it had driven away.

Again, she jumped and again it battered into Jodie.

Sherry knew that checking on her friend this time would do no good.

She started to run.

The car was coming back for another try. She had to get off the road.

It barreled into Jodie again.

This time Sherry got the license number as it drove off — TF 256. She watched to see if it turned around. It didn't. She got back on the highway and walked toward Jodie's body.

There were no moans. No breaths. No nothing. Sherry started to cry. To sob. The sobs racked her body.

A car was coming.

Help.

No. The same car. Getting closer.

Bearing down on her.

She panicked.

She ran down the middle of the highway.

It hit her.

She flew through the air, but she was awake. She was alive. All she had to do was land safely. She was a gymnast. She ought to be able to do that.

She tried.

The road hit her harder than any gym floor ever had. She tried to roll. She did. Off the highway. Into the ditch. And passed out.

TF two five six, she said to herself. Over and over again.

TF two five six.

Two five six.

A police car found her less than ten minutes later. First they had seen Jodie's body. She was dead. Then they found Sherry.

She was awake. She told them what had happened. If it hadn't been for the two battered bodies, they wouldn't have believed her story. It sounded so preposterous.

She even gave them the license plate number.

Half an hour later, they located the car. It was parked on the side of the road less than three miles away. A man was inside it, sitting in the driver's seat, sleeping.

They woke him up and arrested him.

His name was Ted Faber. TF. The car was his. TF 256.

The cops did not believe his story at all. He could not have been asleep and done what he did. He must have been drunk. Or on coke or something.

They took him to the hospital.

He had no alcohol on his breath. Or in his urine. Or blood. Or any other drugs. Just an elevated cholesterol level, which reflected the consumption of too many pizzas over too many years.

Ted Faber's lawyer was not even sure he believed the story but sent him to see both a neurologist and a psychiatrist. I was the neurologist. We both found Ted Faber to be normal. A happily married man who worked too hard but otherwise seemed fine — not the profile of someone who had committed a premeditated murder, or at least willful manslaughter. He was remorseful. He doubted that the girl had lied. He just had no idea why he had done it. And had no memory of having done it. None at all.

We studied him in our sleep lab, doing all-night monitoring of his EEG to see if there were any abnormalities. After all, the incident had occurred during sleep. His study was normal.

We did it for a second night.

Again it was normal.

And a third night, but this time we suddenly startled him less than an hour after he fell asleep. Why not? That was what had occurred on that highway halfway between Rockford and Chicago.

He jumped up in bed.

He cursed.

He looked around.

He yanked off the electrodes, got up, and wandered down the hall. The technician saw him and tried to stop him.

She couldn't.

She tried to waken him.

She couldn't.

She tried to get him to go back to bed.

He wouldn't.

Instead, he wandered from room to room. Opening and slamming doors. Throwing furniture around.

Then he stopped and stood still.

She led him back to bed, and he immediately went back to sleep.

We had the answer. Ted Faber was not a murderer.

When he had been startled in the sleep lab and gotten out of bed, he had been neither asleep nor awake, but somewhere in between. His brain-wave tests had shown that. Normally, sudden arousal is accompanied by a quick switch from sleep activities or sleep waves to the wave patterns that characterize normal wakefulness. Not so in Ted Faber. He had not fully awakened. He had been sidetracked into a state that is called sleep drunkenness. It's a disorder that has been known for centuries but of which there was little, if any, understanding prior to the advent of all-night EEG studies.

Attacks of sleep drunkenness can include unusual and violent behavior, but whatever the behavior, all of the episodes share certain stereotypical features. Without these it is very hard to make a diagnosis. The episodes occur on awakening, never as part of falling asleep, and each episode usually starts following sudden, forced arousal, not as a sequel to spontaneous waking up. This is what happened to Ted Faber, both on the roadside and in the sleep laboratory. Jodie's banging on the car window had suddenly disrupted his sleep. The arousal that precipitates such an episode usually occurs during early deep sleep, most often within ninety minutes of the onset of sleep. Just when Jodie had disrupted him.

In many instances, the sleep has been exceptionally deep owing to excessive fatigue, sleep deficit, or consumption of some alcohol or sedatives. Ted was exhausted and had been for weeks.

The behavior on arousal is usually a quick, immediate, and impulsive response. It is unmotivated, and although it includes normal behaviors like driving a car, this normal behavior is not part of a normal, purposeful response to the situation.

The entire spell is short. Minutes, not hours. And if there is violence associated with it, that violence is senseless. The victim was whoever happened to be present; often it was the person who caused the arousal.

And, of course, the aroused individual has amnesia for what he did. He may, when told what happened, come to believe that he did it and be depressed and remorseful, but he has no recall that he did it.

That fit Ted Faber to a T.

And the EEG proved it. In sleep drunkenness, instead of going from a state of normal sleep to a state of complete arousal, the brain only partially awakens. Part remains asleep. Not everything has slipped into gear. And that was what Ted Faber's EEG had shown just before he pulled off the electrodes. He was awake and responding to his environment, but his cerebral cortex was still asleep. He was awake enough to carry out simple motor acts, even fairly complicated ones, such as removing the electrodes or driving a car, but sophisticated mental behavior involving perception and judgment were arrested.

He did not respond to Jodie's voice.

Or the sleep technician's.

In one case he found himself in a car so he drove it, in the other, in a strange laboratory in which he wandered around slamming doors and throwing furniture.

Then in a few minutes it was over and he went back to sleep.

Ted's lawyers presented the evidence to the state's attorney. All charges should be dropped. After all, Ted was not the first person to carry out an act of violence during such a state. There was precedent for not prosecuting him, precedent that dated back several hundred years.

In the year 1600, a German knight named J. v. Gutlingen was awakened from a state of deep sleep by a friend and companion-at-arms. He awoke in a confused state, and in his confusion, he attacked his friend and stabbed him to death. Gutlingen was tried by the court of Würtemberg and suffered capital punishment. Colonel Culpeper, in England, later in the seventeenth century, fared better. In 1686, this gentleman shot a guardsman and his horse on night patrol. Tried at the Old Bailey, he argued successfully that he was still asleep while committing the crime. The verdict was manslaughter while insane. These two cases are probably the earliest known ones in which violent acts without apparent motivation were committed during the twilight state between sleep and full awakening.

The first fully recorded case of impulsive acting out on arousal occurred in Silesia in 1791. A thirty-two-year-old laborer named Bernard Schidmaizig was awakened from deep sleep around midnight by a noise. He saw the dim outline of a human shape. In a state of apparent terror, he grabbed an ax and hit the terrifying figure. The figure, unfortunately, was his wife and he killed her. After the murder, his mind cleared and he was found embracing his dead wife and crying, "Susanne, wake up!" He was described as a healthy though irritable person, well adjusted in marriage, and a moderate drinker. In his defense, a professor of law, J. F. Meister, argued that there was no rational motive for this act, and that the accused was not fully awake at the time of the murder. He also stated that this homicide was committed in a condition called "sleep drunkenness." He pointed out that a person still sleeping had no free will. Schidmaizig was acquitted.

The first English case involved a woman, Esther Griggs, who in 1859 threw her baby out a window, evidently in an attempt to save the child, when she dreamt that the house was on fire. A passing constable had been virtually an eyewitness to the incident and gave a convincing account of it to a grand jury, who refused to indict her; thus her case did not come to trial.

The state's attorney was not interested in ancient history. He had a dead sixteen-year-old girl on his hands. But he was willing to listen to the medical evidence and have his own expert review the sleep study. The expert did and came to the same conclusion: sleep drunkenness. All charges were dropped.

Ted Faber is still a busy tax lawyer, a good husband, and a loving father. But he makes sure he sleeps in his own bed whenever possible and gets seven or eight hours of sleep each night no matter what. But somehow celebrating his daughter's birthday is no longer the same. And it never will be.

CHAPTER TEN

The Woman Who Had Difficulty Falling

No poet ever interpreted nature as freely as a lawyer interprets law.
— Jean Giradoux

Or a patient his symptoms.

The scenario is all too familiar. A seventy-year-old woman is walking down the street. It is a nice day. There is no wind. No ice. No rain. Suddenly, without any warning, she falls.

And cannot get up.

The ambulance takes her to the hospital. There she is seen by a specialist in emergency medicine. The diagnosis is obvious — a broken hip. The natural progression is almost predetermined.

The patient is immediately carted off to radiology for an X ray and a radiologist to read it. Then to some orthopedic surgeon to have the hip injury evaluated to see what sort of surgical procedure is indicated.

An internist is called in to clear the patient for surgery.

Then an anesthesiologist.

And finally off to the O.R. for the surgery. But the litany doesn't end there.

Postoperatively, the woman is seen again by the internist, who does what he can to prevent a pulmonary embolus and other postop complications.

Next up comes somebody from physical medicine and rehabilitation to encourage early ambulation.

Postoperatively the patient may also be seen by an endocrinologist or rheumatologist to see why her bones broke so easily. Does she have osteoporosis? Can anything be done to prevent further breaks?

But far too often no one has asked the key question: why did she fall?

That to me is what differentiates the neurologist from all other physicians. A patient falls and breaks her hip, and everyone else worries about fixing that hip as quickly as possible and preventing any complications or further breaks.

Only the neurologist remembers to ask why she fell.

The neurologist, and sometimes the cardiologist. For falling belongs to these specialties. From the point of view of the specialists, a patient falls for one of two reasons. Either the heart does not get sufficient blood to the brain, and as a result the patient faints, or the brain or some other part of the nervous system isn't working right.

Those are the choices.

Once a cardiac cause has been ruled out, there is a long list of possible neurological explanations: gait imbalance, cerebellar disease, impaired balance reflexes from Parkinson's disease, abnormal movements, and especially seizures — the falling sickness.

Mrs. Anastasia Trosky was referred to me because of falling. Or as she put it, with her Slavic accent, "Falling. I have difficulty with it. Difficulty falling, doctor." She hoped she was in the right place. None of the other doctors had helped her. Could I?

I had no idea. I had not taken her history. Nor had I examined her. But she was in the right place. I assured her I often examined patients who had falling difficulties.

She was sixty-four when I saw her for that first, last, and only time. She looked closer to seventy-four. She was just over five feet two and weighed perhaps one hundred and thirty-five pounds, although it was hard to tell since she never took off her long, dark raincoat. Or her babushka. Or her sunglasses. It was only early April, and there was very little sunlight in my examining room.

When I asked her about the glasses, she merely said that she always wore them.

Why?

Because she felt better that way.

Occasionally patients with seizures are very sensitive to light, and sudden bright flashes can cause seizures. Wearing sunglasses doesn't really prevent that, but some patients somehow feel safer wearing them. The belief in amulets dies hard.

"What seems to be the problem?" I asked.

For ten years she had had lightninglike jerks of her body.

How did they start?

Like a shot out of the blue.

Did she ever get a warning?

She thought for a moment and then said, "Never."

Many seizure patients have warnings or auras. "Did," I continued, "the jerks last very long?"

"No, no," I was told. They were very brief. Brief. They were over almost before they began. Seconds at the most.

Myoclonus, I said to myself. Repetitive myoclonic jerks. Such jerks can be light-sensitive, and if the legs were involved could result in falls. And injuries. Myoclonic seizures. Perhaps an EEG would document her seizures and their precipitation by light.

"What jerks?" I asked.

"Everything," she said.

I asked her to be more specific.

She was.

Her head. Her arms. Her legs. Her trunk. "Everything," she concluded.

"How often does it happen?"

"All the time. Constantly."

I was surprised by this response, since I had not yet seen so much as a minor twitch, much less a massive jerk. "All the time?"

"Whenever I walk."

"So you must fall a lot."

"No. Not yet. I've been very lucky."

I had her walk for me.

No sooner did she stand up than one of her jerks hit her. Her head flew back, but not too far. Both arms flung out, one up and one down. Her left leg kicked forward, and her right leg stayed planted very firmly.

She swayed.

Back and forth.
She tipped to the right.
Then to the left.
Back and forth.
Swaying her hips.
And counterbalancing each hip movement by adjusting her outstretched arms.

No tightrope walker had ever displayed better balance. Or been less likely to fall. But had that not been what she had said to me? "Difficulty falling?" She had been absolutely right. She not only had difficulty falling; for her, falling bordered on the impossible.

Then her left leg came down and she took a step.
Followed by a second one.
And a third.
Then it struck again.

But it was entirely different. This time her right leg lifted. As did her right arm. While her left leg stayed firm on the floor and her left arm flailed purposefully to counter her hip movement.

Overall I watched about a dozen such episodes. No two were the same. The parade of gesticulations varied from episode to episode. They were not the stereotypical jerks of myoclonic seizures. An EEG would be of no help. Yet, I realized, in a strange way they were all identical. Mrs. Trosky's episodes were not neurological at all. Not myoclonic. Not any kind of seizure. Not chorea. Not dyskinesia. But the sudden kinds of jerks that had their origin in some form of psychiatric distress, not the result of any sort of neurological dysfunction at all. The only neurologist who could help her was Freud, and he, unfortunately, was no longer accepting new patients. The movements carefully disrupted and then maintained her balance. They never really threatened her stability. She had been absolutely correct in her own assessment of her problem. Indeed, she had a great deal of trouble falling.

I went back to my office and called the referring physician and told him my opinion. His name was Dick Etten. He was a former student of mine.

"That can't be," he said.

"Why not?" I countered.

"She's been published. She's had these attacks for years. She was seen by a cardiovascular surgeon. He found a kink in her carotid artery."

"Those are always meaningless," I commented.

"He operated on her and she got better and he published her history, X ray, and the surgical results." Etten even gave me the reference. It had been published by a prestigious surgical journal.

"But she's crazy."

"I always thought so. And now her attacks are back, and he wants to operate again."

"She's sixty-four! And crazy."

"I know," he agreed.

"Should I tell her that she shouldn't have surgery?" I asked him.

"No, she won't believe you. Send me a letter."

I did as he requested and thought that that was the end of the story.

It was not a unique story at all. Physicians have been fooled before. And will be again.

My problem was whether or not to write a letter publicly repudiating the surgeon who had claimed to have cured this woman's seizurelike attacks by operating on a kinked blood vessel. If I didn't, some other surgeon might well make the same kind of mistake.

I started the letter, trying not to be too sarcastic. It was difficult.

I heard from Dick Etten about two months later. He wanted me to see Mrs. Trosky again.

She had gone back to the same cardiovascular surgeon. After all, the surgeon had helped her before and he was certain he could help her again. The neurologists certainly hadn't helped her.

He operated on her carotid artery on the other side. It too was kinked.

She got no better.

And now her face felt as if a rat was gnawing on it.

"She's crazy," I said.

"I know. But he shouldn't have operated on her."

"The technical term is surgical mayhem. I won't be able to help her."

"What should I do?"

"Keep her away from other surgeons."

"I'm trying."

I wrote a second letter to the editor. It suffered the same fate as my first letter about Mrs. Trosky, the one I had sent to Dick Etten, telling him that she didn't need surgery. No one had paid much attention to that letter, either.

I heard about Mrs. Trosky one more time. From a malpractice attorney. He was contemplating a suit against the cardiovascular surgeon.

Was the surgery indicated?

No.

Then he had a case.

I was skeptical.

Why?

There was no way that carotid surgery could cause facial pain.

Was I certain?

Yes.

So why did she have the pain?

She was a hysteric in the classical sense; she converted some unresolved psychiatric difficulty into a medical symptom of flamboyant character. Where was Freud when I needed him?

Was I saying she was crazy? That the unneeded stress of surgery had tipped her over the edge?

"Not at all," I insisted. Her hysteria had come first. That was why she had difficulty falling in the first place, I reminded him. "And," I concluded, "the concept that adding a new hysterical complaint to the repertoire of somebody who is already as hysterical as the day is long would be causing harm to that person should be laughed out of court."

"But she is in pain," he countered.

"Just like she falls," I replied.

"But you told me that she never really falls."

"I rest my case. Or rather your case."

CHAPTER ELEVEN

Not Tonight, Dear

Niagara Falls is only the second biggest disappointment of the standard honeymoon.

— Oscar Wilde
(1854–1900)

Something was wrong. Georgia Luks had never had headaches in her entire life. Her mother had headaches. Every month, with her periods. And her father's mother, Grandma Luks, had headaches all the time. But Georgia couldn't recall the last time she'd had a headache. Perhaps she'd had one in high school. But she had now had this one for almost a week. It had begun as a dull ache behind her left eye. It was not really painful at first. Just enough of an ache so that she knew it was there. But that ache never went away, and each day it got worse. Now it felt as if something was boring into her left eye, from behind the eyeball. It was getting so bad that it was hard for her to concentrate. And even harder to relax.

She had to be more nervous than she imagined. After all, she had a right to be nervous. A girl doesn't get married every day. And she was only going to get married once. One marriage. One headache. A small enough price to pay to spend her life with someone as wonderful as William Glackens.

Why was she so nervous?

She had no idea. It wasn't the old-fashioned reason. She and Bill had been lovers for over a year. They had lived together for the last six months. He was the best lover she had ever had. Kind, considerate, thoughtful, tender, yet strong. She got excited just thinking about him.

No, she certainly wasn't afraid of sex. Nor worried about it.

Except they hadn't made love in four nights now. The headache made it impossible for her to relax. Four consecutive nights. That had never happened before. Bill had been so sweet. He hadn't made any jokes. No sarcasm about "Not tonight, honey, I have a headache." He was such a dear.

"You're just nervous." He had smiled. And then he had said, "Or perhaps you want our wedding night to be special. We'll be in our own villa by the seashore. And we'll make love for the first time in two weeks. Is that it?"

No, she just had a headache.

"Well, make sure it's gone by our wedding night," he had said and then kissed her good night.

That was three nights ago. And the headache wasn't gone. It was still there. Getting worse each day. She talked to her mother about it. It had to be nerves, her mother reassured her.

But what was she nervous about?

The wedding.

But her mother was doing all the planning. Making all the arrangements. And everything was all set. Wasn't it?

It was.

And there were no problems. Were there?

None. Everything would come off without a hitch.

Then why should she be nervous?

"Well, when you're married to a man," her mother began, "he has . . . certain . . . expectations . . . and . . ."

"Mother, we've been making love for over a year. We've been living together for six months. I already know he picks his toes in bed."

Her mother nodded.

"The commitment. Maybe you're afraid of making a commitment."

"I love Bill. I want to have children with him. I want to spend my entire life sharing his bed."

"Maybe you're afraid that might not happen."

"It sure won't if this headache doesn't stop. I . . ." she stopped. It wasn't her mother's business as to whether she and Bill had made love the previous night.

They went on to talk about the wedding. They had talked about everything dozens of times. But that didn't stop her mother. She loved each and every detail. The flowers. The food. The band. Six musicians and a singer. The music. The seating arrangements. That discussion could go on forever and seemed to.

Georgia couldn't stand it. She felt as if her head were going to explode.

Her mother told her that Uncle Carl was going to sit with the Zorachs.

That was too much for Georgia. She exploded. She and her mother had their first argument in years. It was their first fight about the wedding arrangements. The fight lasted less than a minute and left Georgia in tears with her head on her mother's chest.

"You are nervous, dear. Why don't you go upstairs to your old room and sleep here tonight? I'll call Bill. He'll understand."

Georgia did just that. She slept better that night than she had in a week. Perhaps her mom was right. Nerves. Anxiety. However, the next morning, the headache was still there. And worse than ever.

That day she stayed home from work. She talked to Bill on the phone.

He seemed angry.

She had deserted him. And left him alone. And gone back home. It wasn't the sex. He'd already written that off.

Once again she exploded. She wasn't a cold bitch. She wasn't teasing him.

One thing led to another.

Maybe her mother was right. Maybe she was afraid of commitment. Maybe they both were.

Bill hung up.

Georgia was again in tears.

She waited five minutes. Her entire head was throbbing. No. It wasn't her entire head, just the left half of it.

Throbbing.

Pounding.

As if someone were jumping rope behind her left eye.

And not just anyone.

A three-hundred-pound gorilla.

The image made her smile. She called Bill. She apologized. She was just nervous. She'd never gotten married before. She'd never been in love before. And she wanted their life to be so perfect.

So did he. His anger melted away.

She told him about the headaches.

"Go see a doctor," he suggested.

She'd do that.

And she did. She saw their family G.P., Dr. Bierstadt. He was an experienced old-timer who'd been her only doctor from the time she was born. He loved her like a daughter.

"Nerves," he said. "But to be on the safe side, we'll X-ray your sinuses. Could be sinusitis."

The X rays were negative. No sinusitis. He prescribed some Valium. It seemed to help. She went home to Bill. She felt more relaxed. Not enough, but she fell asleep hugging him. That helped.

The next morning, they awoke early. They both knew what they wanted to do. And Bill knew just how to arouse her.

Slowly.

Gently.

Wonderfully.

And she knew just how to arouse him. He'd never felt bigger. Or stronger.

He was above her now. She'd never wanted him more. Never needed him more. Never wanted to please him more. Never wanted to fulfill his needs this much. This was what love was all about, sharing, pleasing, satisfying, giving.

Her head was pounding.

Blasting away.

She didn't care.

He stopped.

"What's wrong?" she asked.

"Your eye."

"My eye?"

"Your left eye."

"What's wrong with my left eye?" she asked. He was no longer ready to enter her. What had she done wrong?

"It's closed."

The throbbing behind her eye was slowing down.

Bill moved away. Together they got out of bed and walked over to the mirror.

Her left eye was closed. The upper eyelid was all the way down. She tried to will it open. Her right eye opened all the way. Her left eye stayed shut. The only way she could open it was by lifting the upper lid with her finger.

"That's not your nerves," Bill said anxiously.

Bill drove her to Dr. Bierstadt's office.

"What's wrong?" Dr. Bierstadt asked.

"I can't open my eye," she answered.

He examined her.

"What's wrong?" she asked.

"You can't open your eye," he answered, adding, "You should see an ophthalmologist."

"Who?"

"Dr. Francis."

Dr. Bierstadt called and made the appointment. Sam Francis would see her the next morning.

That night before she went to bed, Georgia looked in the mirror. Her left eye was completely shut. She lifted her eyelid with her finger. Something else was wrong with her left eye. Her pupil was gigantic. Much larger than the pupil of her right eye.

Why was that?

Had it been that way that morning?

She couldn't remember.

She asked Bill. He couldn't remember, either.

Bill drove her to see Dr. Francis. His office was in Chicago. Downtown. In a new building on North Michigan Avenue.

It was new. And lavish. With lots of modern art. Bright, splashy abstract paintings. One was by De Kooning. She recognized the name. It was an original De Kooning. He had to be a very good doctor.

When she lifted her left eyelid to get a better look, the picture became blurred.

"What's wrong?" Dr. Francis asked her.

"I can't open my eye," Georgia replied. She also told him about her headaches. And the wedding.

He nodded sagely and examined her.

"What's wrong?" she asked.

"You can't open your eye," he began. "You are having a very severe, prolonged migraine."

"Oh," she said, relieved by the diagnosis. She was worried about far more serious matters. A brain tumor. A stroke. A migraine was no big deal. Lots of people had migraines. Her grandmother had them.

He nodded. Migraines are often hereditary, he told her. She told him about Grandma Luks and her headaches, and Dr. Francis nodded again.

"Why can't I open my eye?"

He explained that in migraines, the carotid artery swells. That artery is right behind the eye, just where her pain had started.

She nodded.

"And sometimes that swollen artery presses on some of the small nerves going to the eye, causing the eyelid to droop. And the pupil to get small. It's called Horner's syndrome. It's nothing to worry about. It'll go away."

"When?"

"In a few weeks."

"In time for the wedding?"

"No."

"But it will get better?"

"Yes," he assured her.

"But the pupil is big, not small," she said, a trifle worried.

"Makes no difference," he said. His voice exuded confidence, as did his demeanor, and his office, and his De Kooning.

She told him she liked his art. He did, too. He was especially proud of his De Kooning.

Were any tests necessary?

No.

Could he give her some medicine for the headaches?

He wrote out a prescription.

Was there anything she shouldn't do?

No.

She remembered that her headache got worse when she and Bill had tried to make love.

She asked the doctor.

"No," he said. "No limitations. Have a great honeymoon. You'll be fine."

She already felt better.

Georgia's eye did not get any better. She checked every time she got near a mirror. Her eyelid just would not move. And her pupil stayed wide open. And her vision out of the eye remained blurred. But her headaches were better. They were reduced to just a dull throb. Not really painful anymore. That medicine that Dr. Francis had prescribed was doing the trick.

She asked her friend who was a nurse to look up Horner's syndrome for her. Her friend did. It was usually not anything serious at all. The little nerves going to the eye got injured. The eyelid dropped and the pupil got small.

Small? Was she sure?

That's what the book said.

But hers was big. Dr. Francis had said that sometimes the pupil got big.

That wasn't in her friend's books.

For a moment Georgia got worried, but for only a moment. Dr. Francis was a well-known specialist. And she was getting better. She'd see him again when she got back from her honeymoon. She wanted to see his De Kooning again.

The wedding went off without a hitch. Well, almost without a hitch. The photographer tried hard to take as many profile shots of her as he could. Right profile, of course.

But it was fun.

She took her pills. And ate and danced and drank. And then they raced to the airport and took the last flight out to Acapulco. For ten glorious days. Of sun, beach, and each other. They did not wait very long for each other. It had already been far too long. And Dr. Francis had told her she had nothing to worry about.

Bill, as always, was gentle.

Slow.

Loving.

She could feel her heart pounding.

She was so excited.

It had never been like this.

Her eye began to throb.

To pound.

To blast away.

To explode.

She felt as if her head were going to blow apart.

She wanted Bill to stop.

She tried to tell him to stop.

She opened her mouth.

No words came out.

More pounding.

More throbbing.

More explosions.

She was sick. She was going to vomit.

No.

Not that.

Yes.

She couldn't stop herself.

She retched. Her head snapped forward. Her mouth flew open. She vomited.

Once.

Twice.

A third time.

And then she felt one more explosion.

And nothing else. Nothing else at all.

As soon as she threw up, Bill jumped away and yelled her name.

Georgia never replied. She never responded at all. Bill shook her. Still she didn't reply. She was unconscious. Comatose.

In less than an hour, she was at the hospital. Later that day she was flown to Mexico City. There they made a diagnosis. Georgia Glackens had an aneurysm — a small blister on the carotid artery — just behind her left eye. That was what had caused her headache.

"And the Horner's syndrome," Bill added.

"No, no. She does not have a Horner's syndrome," the neurosurgeon said. "A Horner's means a small pupil. Hers is very big."

Bill just nodded.

And now the aneurysm had burst, spilling blood inside her head and causing some damage to her brain.

How much damage?

The neurosurgeon wasn't sure. But he was sure of two things. She needed an operation to make certain that the aneurysm didn't bleed again. And that it was a tragedy that someone hadn't made the diagnosis sooner, before the aneurysm burst.

The surgery went well. There were no complications. Ten days later, Georgia came back to Chicago. She had a mild degree of weakness of her right arm and right leg, and she was aphasic. Both her right-sided weakness and her speech difficulty reflected damage to her left hemisphere, which had been severely injured by the torrent of blood pumped into it by the rupture of the aneurysm. She never improved very much. She was left with a severe aphasia. Her speech abilities were not much better than those of an average four-year-old.

The case came to trial four years later. I was the expert witness for the plaintiff, Georgia Glackens. At trial, the major role of the expert witness is that of teacher. He must teach the jury what happened. What went wrong. What was done that shouldn't have been done. What wasn't done that should have been done. The errors of commission and the errors of omission, and how these errors injured the plaintiff. The extent of the injury. And its prognosis. It's not much different from teaching medical students.

I started by teaching the jury about the eye. I taught them slowly, in response to a set of prearranged questions. And as I taught, I looked at them, one at a time. For they were the audience. Not Georgia Glackens's lawyer, Tom Benton, who was asking the questions. Two different nerves control the eyelid and the pupil. The first, and less important, is the sympathetic nerve — a group of small fibers that travel along the carotid artery to get to the eye. If this group of fibers is not working adequately, the eyelid droops — but only a few millimeters. It never closes all the way. And the pupil gets smaller. That's called Horner's syndrome — a mild droop and a small pupil.

The other nerve goes directly from the brain stem to the eye. It's called the third cranial nerve. It is the far more important of the two. If it's injured, the upper lid closes and the pupil enlarges, dilates, and no longer gets smaller when light shines in it. As a result, everything looks blurred, the way it does when an ophthalmologist puts drops in your eye to dilate the pupil. That the jury understood. I could tell by the looks on their faces.

"And who," Tom Benton asked, "should know the difference between injury to the third nerve and a Horner's syndrome?"

"Any and every first-year medical student," I replied, looking at him for the first time.

"An ophthalomogist?"

"Of course."

"Did Georgia Luks-Glackens ever have a Horner's syndrome?"

"No."

"Why not?"

I looked back at the jury. It was time to teach them a bit more. Georgia's eyelid was completely closed. Anyone could see that by looking at her wedding pictures. The lawyer had passed those to the jury earlier in the trial. A Horner's syndrome cannot completely close the eye. A third-nerve injury does that. Her pupil was enlarged. A Horner's syndrome causes a small pupil. A third-nerve injury causes a large pupil. Her vision was blurred. A Horner's syndrome cannot do that. A third-nerve injury does.

"Dr. Klawans," Benton began. It was time for the legal formula. "In your opinion, did Dr. Francis deviate from the accepted standard of care?"

"Yes."

"How?"

"His diagnosis of a Horner's syndrome was a deviation from the standard of care."

"Did that deviation from the standard of care harm Mrs. Glackens?"

The big question. I looked back at the jury.

"Yes."

"How?"

"A Horner's syndrome is usually benign. A third-nerve injury is a warning of something far more dangerous, especially if it is associated with pain. A painful third-nerve paralysis. That means an unruptured aneurysm of the carotid artery until proved otherwise. It's a warning. That is a true emergency. That aneurysm must be diagnosed and treated before it ruptures and causes permanent brain injury. Dr. Francis made the wrong diagnosis. As a result, the right diagnosis was never made and Mrs. Glackens is now permanently disabled by right-sided weakness and a terrible speech disability. She talks like a four-year-old. It will affect her entire life. Her work. She was a college graduate. Now she can do only menial jobs. Her interpersonal relationships. If she has a child, that child will outgrow her intellectually in five years."

It was time for the cross-examination. Dr. Francis's lawyer was named Guston. Phil Guston. He really wasn't Francis's lawyer. He was the lawyer for Francis's insurance company. They picked him and paid him, and he reported to them. They called all the shots, not Sam Francis. But you can't even mention them in court. Some system.

His job was to discredit me, which can be done in any number of ways. He could try to prove that what I said was wrong. That is the job of the expert, so on cross-examination they usually attack other aspects of my testimony. Was I really an expert on what Sam Francis should know?

"Dr. Klawans, are you an ophthalomogist?"

"No," I admitted.

"Did you ever take an ophthalmology residency?"

"No."

"Then how can you pretend to be an expert on what ophthalmologists should know about the third nerve and Horner's syndrome?"

I looked him straight in the eye. "I teach them neurology. All ophthalmology residents rotate through neurology. And we neurologists teach them. We know exactly what they should know. That's our job. That's my job. I know."

Strike one. He had made a mistake. He had asked this question blindly, not knowing what the answer would be. It had cost him points. He had embarrassed himself in front of the jury. That was worse than being wrong. He had attacked what he thought was a weakness and found a strength. He had increased my credibility and in so doing decreased his own.

Time for another tactic.

"Dr. Klawans, are you saying that Dr. Francis should have made the diagnosis of a . . . what did you call it . . . an unruptured aneurysm? These must be very rare. How many do you see in a year?"

"One. Perhaps two."

"Very rare. You only see one or two a year and you believe that Dr. Francis, who is not a neurologist, should have been able to make the diagnosis."

"No, sir. I never said that. I said he should not have made the wrong diagnosis. He should have known that there was an injury to the third nerve and that that was an emergency and referred Ms. Luks to either a neurologist or a neurosurgeon. And he certainly should not have made a diagnosis of a Horner's syndrome."

"Because he's an ophthalmologist?"

"No, because he finished his first year in medical school. All first-year medical students know the difference between a third-nerve palsy and Horner's syndrome."

Strike two.

"You are not an expert on headaches, are you?"

"I have written several articles on headaches."

"But by your own admission you are not an expert?"

"My own admission? Not that I know of."

He went back and picked up a book. It was my first novel, *Sins of Commission*. He opened the book.

"Did you write this paragraph?" he asked, and then he read from the book.

"Right. But as they pointed out, that's not true. Most headaches caused by sex are just simple migraines. You know, Klawans is not a headache doctor. He doesn't specialize in headaches, so at a meeting once I asked him how come he wrote that paper. He said he only wrote it because he wanted to write a second paper and send it to some prestigious place like the *New England Journal of Medicine* — a follow-up paper dealing with the therapy of such headaches."

Did you write that?"

"Yes."

"So you wrote, quote, 'Klawans is not a headache doctor. He doesn't specialize in headaches,' unquote."

"Yes."

"But today you are acting as if you are an expert in headaches and that you can tell us what Dr. Francis should have known about Georgia's headaches. Which should we believe, Dr. Klawans? The one you want us to believe today or what you said three years ago?"

He was winning, but he'd given me an opening and I jumped in with both feet, for that's how the game is won. "I never said that."

"It's right here in this book. Do you deny writing this book?"

"No. I wrote the book, and I'm proud of that book. It was a Book-of-the-Month-Club selection. But I never said that. I wrote that."

"What's the difference?"

"I wrote that as a fictional speech by a fictional character. It's fiction."

He'd almost hit a home run, but it had ended up as a long, loud foul. He had one more chance. One last shot. He went back to his table and picked up another book, my second novel, *Informed Consent*.

"You also wrote this novel, didn't you?"

"Yes."

And he started to read from the prologue, in which my hero/ neurologist is an expert witness for a plaintiff in a medical malpractice case.

The lawyer began to read.

Georgia's lawyer objected.

The judge overruled his objection when the defense attorney said that it had to do with my credibility.

Paul had been careful to apportion a smile to each of the jurors as they filed in. He was feeling pretty confident despite the prickly discomfort of his gray worsted testifying suit. Up until a year ago, Paul had consistently made good on his vow

to wear suits only to funerals. But when the lawyers insisted
that the jurors wouldn't believe an expert witness if he weren't
"properly attired," ultimately taking their argument, and
Paul, out shopping, their reluctant witness could only agree to
wear the suit they picked out for him and paid for. Paul
looked down at his feet. He had worn the appropriate shoes
and his socks matched both his tie and each other.

"Did you write that, Dr. Klawans?"
"Yes, sir."
"And you are wearing a suit today, aren't you?"
"Yes."
"Did you buy that suit yourself?"
"Objection."
"I'll withdraw that question."
One point for the bad guys.
He began reading again.

> He had impressed them yesterday. His testimony had gone
> well. He had taken his time and looked at each of them, first
> one and then another, as he had given his expert opinions. It
> was an old trick but to a real pro that kind of technique came
> instinctively. Talking to a jury was not that much different
> from giving a good lecture. To be effective you had to talk to
> each listener as an individual and to the group as a whole at the
> same time.

"You wrote that too, didn't you?"
He smiled at the jury, looking at them one at a time, and then
began to read again:

> The black foreman had liked him. So had the old lady in the
> back row. He was always a hit with the old ladies. Then again,
> he was probably the only witness who had paid any attention
> at all to her. Strange, how it all became a contest. He was an
> expert witness for a woman whose life had been ruined by a
> hack surgeon. As an expert witness he should only be inter-
> ested in the truth, but since he was also concerned with justice
> he did care who won the case. The three-piece suit, the eye

contact, and even the old lady in the back row all were byprod-
ucts of Paul's absolute certainty that Courtney was a butcher
who had damn near killed Mrs. Martin by out and out malpractice.

"You did write all of that, didn't you?"

"Yes, sir."

"So that is what you think your role is as an expert witness? To
win the case? Not just to tell what you think is the truth?"

"No, sir."

"But you wrote those words, didn't you?"

"That book is a novel," I replied, looking toward the jury. "A
work of fiction. Not a scientific article. What you have just read to
me are the fictitious thoughts of a fictitious character in a fictitious
trial. One that never took place."

"Judge," the lawyer said, "I move to have you strike that answer as nonresponsive."

The judge shook his head. "I'll do one better. I'm going to strike
the entire line of questioning as irrelevant."

On redirect, Georgia's attorney followed up one line of questioning. He wanted to get the jury thinking about Georgia, not
about me and my novels. "Mr. Guston," he began, "asked you
about an article you had written about headaches during sexual
activity."

He had to start that way. On redirect, he could only ask me
about subjects that were brought up during cross-examination.

"Yes," I replied.

"Can you tell us about that subject?"

I could and did, knowing just what he wanted. I explained how
severe headaches during intercourse were often due to bleeding
into the brain from a ruptured aneurysm. That the increased heart
rate and blood pressure accompanying such intense activity can
cause an aneurysm to burst.

"Is that what happened to Georgia?"

"Yes."

"Is that a known risk of an undiagnosed aneurysm?"

"Yes."

"If the correct diagnosis had been made and the aneurysm had been treated, could she have gotten married and gone on her honeymoon and made love to her husband without that happening?"

"Yes."

"I have no further questions."

That night the insurance company settled the case for one and a half million dollars, which was the limit of Dr. Francis's insurance policy. Georgia's attorney called to give me the news. The insurance company's only hope had been to destroy my credibility. Their own expert witnesses were very weak and would probably not have stood up under cross-examination. Destroying me was their only hope. Not what I said necessarily, but me. Had I crumbled, the case would have settled for a million. But I hadn't crumbled. So Georgia got one and a half million.

"One point five million," I commented.

"Not bad."

"Yeah. She can almost buy a nice De Kooning for that. Not a great one. Not *Woman One* or *Woman Two*, but a nice one."

"Why would she want a De Kooning?" he asked.

"She wouldn't," I said. "Believe me, she wouldn't."

CHAPTER TWELVE

The Twinkie Defense

Dan White and the Murder of the Mayor of San Francisco

Judges and juries should determine issues of guilt and innocence, sanity and insanity . . . psychiatrists are often pushed
into making that decision for them. There is a tendency for
psychiatrists to find mental illness in every instance of emotional stress. I personally resist this.

> — Martin Blinder, M.D., *psychiatrist,*
> *who acted as an expert witness for*
> *the defense. Quoted by D. Wegers in*
> *the* San Francisco Chronicle,
> *May 24, 1979.*

There was clearly some sort of a deal not to hit on the political
aspects of this case. Everybody in town knew from the early
defense subpoenas — for most every politician in town — that
this was going to be a political trial. The defense was going to
show the tensions — gays, liberals, the changes in town —
that were offending Dan White's sense of values. But the defense dropped that aspect of its case. That's why the trial
ended much earlier than expected. There had to be some sort
of "you don't get rough, we don't get rough" understanding
worked out.

> — Jack Webb, *a*
> *member of the City*
> *Charter Commision.*
> *Quoted by Warren Hinckle in the*
> San Francisco Chronicle, *May 23,*
> *1979.*

The facts of the crimes were never in doubt. No one actually
disputed them. Not at trial, nor before, nor afterward. In October
of 1978, Dan White, who had previously been a policeman in San

Francisco, resigned from his position as a city supervisor. The reason he gave for his resignation was that his salary of $9,000 was not enough for him to support his wife and their infant. That seems reasonable and logical enough; $9,000 was not much of an annual income, considering the cost of living in San Francisco in 1978. But Dan White soon had a change of heart. He decided that he wanted his job back, so he asked Mayor George Moscone to reappoint him. The mayor's initial reaction was positive. White could have his old job back and once again be a city supervisor at $9,000 per year. But then the mayor changed his mind. Dan White could not have his job back. On November 27, 1978, Dan White took his gun and some extra ammunition and went to City Hall, arriving there just one hour before Mayor Moscone was to announce the name of the new supervisor who was to take Dan White's old job. Dan White did not enter City Hall through the main entrance with its guards and metal detectors. Instead, he entered through a large window in the basement. He then went straight to Mayor Moscone's office and shot the mayor four times. White then reloaded the gun and went to Harvey Milk's office and shot him five times. In both instances, the victims were first shot in their bodies, and then, after they were on the floor, were each shot twice in the head.

Those were the facts. Two simple cases of premeditated, first-degree murder. Why premeditated?

How could it be otherwise? White took his gun and extra bullets. He avoided the metal detectors. He executed his victims. And he had a personal motive. The mayor was not going to give him his job back, and Harvey Milk had been instrumental in convincing the mayor not to, a fact that Dan White knew. And his motive may have gone even deeper. At the time, Harvey Milk was the only publicly avowed homosexual in public office in the U.S. Mayor Moscone was friendly toward the large, politically active homosexual community of San Francisco. White not only had a personal motive based on a single discussion, he may also have had a far more deep-seated and politically explosive motive, relating to Harvey Milk's homosexuality and White's own attitudes toward that and the growing political power of the homosexual community of San Francisco.

Could it have been a murder born out of hatred? Out of some sort of homophobia?

Could it have been, in the true sense, a political murder?

Either of these possibilities could have become an explosive issue especially in San Francisco, especially in 1979.

But none of these issues ever came up at the trial.

In May 1979, White, charged with two counts of first-degree murder, was tried in San Francisco. He pleaded "not guilty by reason of diminished responsibility."

Diminished responsibility under California law has a very specific meaning, which is defined in the instructions given to the jury:

> "If you find from the evidence that at the time the alleged crime was committed, the defendant had substantially reduced mental capacity, whether caused by mental illness, mental defect, intoxication, or any other cause, you must consider what effect, if any, this diminished capacity had on the defendant's ability to form any of the specific mental states that are essential elements of murder and voluntary manslaughter."

This contrasts with first-degree murder, in which the murderer must have carried out an unlawful killing with "malice aforethought," in other words, premeditation or planning. Like taking extra ammunition and avoiding metal detectors.

The defense hired four psychiatrists and one psychologist to act as expert witnesses. All five came to the same conclusion. Dan White could not have carried out a premeditated, first-degree murder because he had "diminished capacity." He was not capable of such premeditation, such planning, such malice aforethought.

Why not?

He had a psychiatric disease.

What disease?

Recurrent attacks of depression.

This theme was expressed by all of the defense experts in their direct testimony when answering questions asked by the defense attorney, Douglas Schmidt. The answer of Dr. Donald Lunde to the question as to whether Dan White suffered from mental illness at the time of the crime is typical of the opinions of all five experts.

"My opinion is that he (White) was suffering from mental illness on or prior to November 27, 1978. The mental illness is depression of a fairly severe degree; secondarily, he also has, of long-standing duration, a very compulsive personality . . . that is someone who, from a fairly early age, is quite rigid, overly conscientious, overly upset, uptight as an adult, characterized as workaholic . . . I think that probably those are genetic, biochemical factors that contribute to depression of this sort . . ."

Lunde also denied any premeditation on White's part.

"And in Mr. White's case, he not only did not premeditate or deliberate these killings, but as a result of his mental condition, he was not capable of any kind of mature, meaningful reflection on the morning of November 27, 1978, of last year."

Schmidt also asked Lunde if White had harbored malice against the victims. Lunde answered:

". . . at the time of these killings (White) was not thinking about the effect of his behavior on human life, the value of human life . . . The last thing he was doing, capable of doing, was thinking clearly about his obligations to society, other people, the law, and so on."

The defense replaced premeditation with malice aforethought with a far different state of mind — that of depression.

But was that enough? Everyone gets depressed from time to time. Everyone knows people who have been depressed. They haven't gone out and killed anyone. Certainly not the ones who precipitated the depression. It's not much of a leap from believing that White was so depressed by Moscone's refusal to rehire him that he shot both Moscone and Milk, the guy who had persuaded the mayor to replace him, because he was depressed, to imagining that he was more angry than depressed. More pissed off than unhappy. And that he went out and killed those SOBs. You didn't have to be a board-certified psychiatrist to understand such behavior.

Such premeditated behavior.

With malice aforethought.

Enter yet another defense expert, another psychiatrist, Dr. Martin Blinder.

Blinder maintained that White suffered from mental illness not only when he shot Moscone and Milk but all of his adult life. He diagnosed White's illness as a "manic-depressive syndrome dating back to adolescence," and attributed this illness to a biochemical defect in his body.

"White's frequent episodes of depression," Blinder told the jury, "were escalated by an exclusive diet of junk food — Twinkies, cupcakes and Cokes. . . ."

Blinder noted that whenever White felt things were not going right, he would abandon his usual regimen of good nutrition, in which he combined healthful foods with a program of vigorous exercise, and go off on high-sugar, junk-food binges. Typically, he would sit or lie around, gorging himself with Twinkies and Cokes. According to Blinder, the more junk food White consumed, the worse he seemed to feel psychologically. And again according to Blinder, White would respond to any growing depression by ever greater consumption of such food substitutes. Finally, after several days, he would pull himself together and stop gorging; then and only then, would he begin to feel better, and return to exercising, perhaps even jogging. He would become less inclined to eat junk foods and would be rewarded by an ever-improved mood, and so on. In this way, he cycled back toward a normal mood.

Blinder has given his version of the event preceding the two "murders."

"On November 14, White saw the mayor and told him he had changed his mind and that he wanted his letter of resignation back. The mayor responded by telling him that 'our political differences aside, Dan, you've always given me a fair shake, you're an honest man, and if you come back tomorrow I'll have your letter for you,' which he did. He promised Mr. White reappointment and told the media the same thing. A few days later, however, he told Mr. White that there was a problem, a problem that could be alleviated if White could provide the mayor's office with a show of support for reappointment. Mr. White made sure that this was forthcoming, but by the end of the week, the mayor apparently had pulled back on his previous promise. The mayor's press agent, Mel Wax, told the media, 'The only one who supports Dan White for reappointment is Dan White.' "

This turn of events was apparently quite upsetting to Mr. White, and, according to Blinder, White turned to junk food for solace. White's sister, Nancy, reported to Blinder that Dan White had her bring him two packages of chocolate cupcakes and eight candy bars and a six-pack of Coke. Soon he was planted in front of the TV for hours on end, binging on Twinkies and Cokes. White could not sleep and retreated to the living room couch so that his tossing and turning could not disturb his wife. Unable to sleep at night, he was fatigued and lethargic all day. He felt increasingly despondent, even dazed and confused. He had crying spells, became quite irritable, and wanted to be left alone.

On November 23, late in the evening, news reporter Barbara Taylor called White for "his comment on the fact that he was not gong to be reappointed." This was the first definitive news Mr. White had gotten. He became more distressed, and he didn't sleep that entire night, instead sitting around, his head aching, "drinking copious quantities of soda pop and eating high-sugar cupcakes and candy bars."

This then became the defense. White was not pissed off and out for vengeance. He did not have a major grudge against Moscone and Milk, nor any long-standing hatred or prejudice. He was depressed. Depression is a biochemical disorder of the brain. But White was not just depressed; he was also intoxicated. And such intoxication can be and is a legitimate cause of *diminished capacity*.

Blinder concluded his testimony by telling the jury that there was a lot of recent scientific evidence that demonstrated that physiological aberrations could be caused by the consumption of noxious food substitutes by susceptible individuals. He told them that there were cases in the literature of people who reacted violently after consuming large quantities of refined sugar. Furthermore, there were studies of cerebral allergic reactions to the chemicals that are found in such highly processed foods; some studies had even documented a marked reduction in violent and antisocial behavior in "career criminals" upon the elimination of these substances from their diet, as well as the production of rage reactions in susceptible individuals when challenged by the offending food substances. "For those reasons," he testified, "I would suggest a repeat electroencephalogram preceded by a glucose-tolerance test, as well as a clinical challenge of Mr. White's mental functions with known food antigens, in a controlled setting."

On May 21, 1979, the jury brought in a verdict of voluntary manslaughter. On July 3, 1979, White was given the maximum sentence for his offense — seven years and eight months in prison. With time off for good behavior and for the time he spent in jail awaiting trial, White would be eligible for parole in less than five years.

Why had this been their verdict? Why not plain old-fashioned murder?

In part, because none of the other issues was raised. Contemporary news coverage documented this. According to those stories, some jurors questioned why the prosecution called only one psychiatrist, while the defense called four of them and one psychologist. Other jurors wondered out loud whether the prosecution could find only one such expert witness to speak against White. Jurors said the psychiatric testimony presented by the defense was persuasive, while that of Dr. Roland Levy, the prosecution witness who interviewed White hours after he killed Moscone and Milk, was weak and had been nullified by the cross-examination.

One juror said that the "homosexual issue wasn't raised. And no politics entered into the deliberations. It centered on the condition of White at the time." The same juror added that "the psychiatric testimony was highly influential. It was mainly what we based the verdict on." Concerning the role of junk food in the crime, another juror said: "Some people believed it. Some people didn't. I don't know that much about it. It's new research."

Why had the jurors been allowed to believe Martin Blinder when he told them that White's compulsive diet of candy bars, cupcakes, and Cokes was evidence of a deep depression — "and a source of excessive sugar that had aggravated a chemical imbalance in his brain"? For that is why White got off with manslaughter and not premeditated murder. The Twinkie defense, a defense that was never attacked.

The prosecution used only one expert. He was a psychiatrist, but he was not an expert in biological psychiatry, that section of psychiatry which focuses on the biological or biochemical basis of human behavior.

For the Twinkie defense would have been easy to demolish. Mere child's play. It is not the product of scientific research, but of pseudoscience. It is not that there is little data to support the notion that in susceptible individuals (whatever that means) junk food causes diminished capacity. There are no data. There never have been. What passes for data are anecdotes and apocrypha, not controlled scientific studies. Yes, depression is a biochemical disorder, but Twinkie consumption has never been shown to make it worse and cause diminished capacity. But the testimony was never attacked.

Why not?

It was clear to several observers that more than just the defense helped protect Dan White. San Francisco newspapermen smelled a fish.

Charles McCabe, *San Francisco Chronicle* columnist, wrote: "White had all the old-fashioned prejudices and bigotries. He hated blacks and 'queers' and made no secret of it. . . . The man (Moscone) who double-crossed him had offended his manhood. Moreover, the mayor was the most powerful friend the homosexuals had in this city."

Herb Caen, another *Chronicle* columnist, was equally candid:

> "What's wrong with San Francisco?" was being asked again yesterday . . . one can kill, twice, complete with coup de grace, and get away with it. The grateful defendant was a staunch defender of law and order . . . a religious man who went straight to church after he killed. This is a city of undercurrents, not all of them well hidden. Many police made an open secret of their support for Dan White and their dislike (understatement) of homosexuals . . .

Warren Hinckle, also writing in the *Chronicle,* pulled no punches about his claim that defense and prosecution collaborated

in the depoliticization of the White case — indeed, in White's very
defense. Without some of his observations, the story of the White
affair would be significantly incomplete. He wrote:

". . . when Dan White surrendered his death weapon, the assassin was met at City Prison, according to an eyewitness, with a
reception not inconsistent with that fit for a hero."

One eyewitness to this outrage was White's jailer, the former
undersheriff of San Francisco, James Derman. He was not called as
a witness for the prosecution. Derman told Hinckle, "The attitude
of most of the cops I witnessed seemed to be that Dan White had
done something they were not unhappy about. . . . There is a
profound paranoia about gays in the police department."

Hinckle also quoted, and agreed with, the opinion of Jack
Webb, a member of the City Charter Commission and a former
San Francisco policeman, that

> there was clearly some sort of a deal not to hit on the political
> aspects of this case. Everybody in town knew from the early
> defense subpoenas — for most every politician in town — that
> this was going to be a political trial. The defense was going to
> show the tensions — gays, liberals, the changes in town —
> that were offending Dan White's sense of values. But the de-
> fense dropped that aspect of its case. That's why the trial
> ended much earlier than expected. There had to be some sort
> of "you don't get rough, we don't get rough" understanding
> worked out.

It wasn't just the newsmen who were surprised. Fifteen minutes
after the jury announced its decision, San Francisco Mayor Dianne
Feinstein reacted to the verdict with "disbelief." "As far as I am
concerned, these were two murders," she said.

So why did it come to pass?

I don't know.

Some critics, especially Dr. Thomas Szasz, argued that the ju-
dicial and medical authorities in the Dan White case acted in concert to declare that the crime was not "political" but "psychiatric."
He believes that prosecution and defense cooperated — should one
say "colluded"? — in depoliticizing the assassination. As defense

attorney Stephen Scherr explained to the San Francisco *Examiner* after the trial: "The defense was wary of having gays serve on the jury." He said the attorneys feared that a gay might believe that the slaying of Milk, San Francisco's first openly homosexual supervisor, was a political assassination committed to block gay power. Scherr said such a belief would be contrary to the facts in the case. The prosecution went along with this tactic — which was like excluding black jurors from the trial of the accused assassin of Martin Luther King on the grounds that they might mistakenly believe that the killing had something to do with the fact that King was black.

Why was it done? Was it done to defuse a politically sensitive issue, as a sort of political plea bargaining?

Such questions cannot be answered, but some questions can.

Is the Twinkie defense a legitimate defense?

To my knowledge, it has never again been used successfully.

Was it attacked with appropriate experts?

No.

If the Twinkies caused Dan White to have diminished capacity and kill people, didn't the families of the victim have a case against the manufacturers of Twinkies?

They sure did. All they would have had to prove was that the Twinkies caused White to act with diminished capacity. And not beyond a benefit of a doubt, but just more probably than not.

But no case was ever brought to court.

Why not?

The reader can decide that issue.

AUTHOR'S NOTE

Both sides of the Dan White case can be found in Vol. II, *The American Journal of Forensic Psychiatry* (1981–1982). The specific articles are:

Thomas Szasz, "The Political Use of Psychiatry in the United States: The Case of Dan White." II, 1–11.

Martin Blinder, "My Psychiatric Examination of Dan White." II, 12–22.

George F. Solomon, "Comments on the Case of Dan White." II, 22–26.

Since this is a court case, the reader should have access to all of the testimony. Perhaps someday that will be true. It isn't as I write this. The records have been impounded to protect someone or something. That thing is unlikely to be either truth or justice.

CHAPTER THIRTEEN

"Nobody Shot Me"

The Saga of an Iatrogenic* Disease Told in Three
Suits and an Epilogue

When the police arrived at the garage on Clark Street where
the St. Valentine's Day Massacre had just taken place, one
of the victims was still alive. He was Frank Gusenberg, one of
the last remaining members of the then all but extinct Bugs
Moran gang.

"Who shot you?" the cops asked.

"Nobody shot me," Frank informed them.

SUIT ONE

T.D. or Not T.D.?
That is the question.

In medical school, I never saw a patient with Huntington's chorea. I read a bit about the disease, as I did about many other
neurological disorders. But since Huntington's is not a very common disorder, the space devoted to it in the textbooks I studied
was rather meager. The low incidence of the disorder, combined
with the tendency of many patients with the disease to stay as far
away from medical centers as possible, accounted for this gap in
my medical training. I never saw a patient with tardive dyskinesia,
either. Nor did I ever read about tardive dyskinesia. Neither of

* Iatrogenic: Caused by a physician's treatment of a patient.

these facts is at all surprising, for tardive dyskinesia had not even been invented yet.

All of this began to change during my internship. That was when I first saw a patient with Huntington's chorea. One just happened to be admitted to my floor on a night when I was the intern on call. So I worked him up. And since Huntington's is rather rare, and this was the first such patient admitted to that particular hospital in two years, it was decided that that patient should be presented at medical Grand Rounds; since he was my patient and since I was interested in neurology and since Huntington's chorea was a neurological disease, the powers that be decided that I should be the one to discuss the case. It was up to me to tell everyone everything there was to know about Huntington's chorea.

That was in 1962 and fortunately, for me at least, not much was known about Huntington's chorea then. I didn't appreciate that fact as I spent all my free time in the library wading through every article I could find, starting with Huntington's original description, published some ninety years earlier. It was only as I finished my survey that I realized how brilliantly George Huntington, a general practitioner with no training in the field of neurology and with no understanding at all of the as yet undiscovered field of genetics, had analyzed his patients and their histories. Huntington recognized all of the salient features of the disease that now bears his name. The onset was usually during adult life, most frequently during the thirties or forties. The disease included abnormal involuntary movements and a wide diversity of psychiatric symptoms varying from agitation and depression to severe psychosis. But the most important characteristic was the strictly hereditary nature of the disorder. Huntington realized that if a parent had the disease, his or her children could develop the disorder. On the other hand, if the offspring of an affected individual reached forty or fifty without having developed the disease, his or her children could neither develop nor transmit the disease. That was all Huntington knew. In 1962, we didn't really know much more. So at Grand Rounds, I talked more about the history of the disease and its ravages over the centuries, than about the disease itself. After all, there was little to discuss clinically. There were virtually no related disorders to discuss.

Nothing else produced such movements in adults. There was no differential diagnosis.

In the next ten years, all that changed.

Today, we have more diseases that we have to differentiate from Huntington's chorea. And one of these is tardive dyskinesia, unfondly referred to by its acronym, T.D. It is, by definition, an iatrogenic disease. The only cause is long-term exposure to drugs used to treat schizophrenia. These antipsychotic agents belong to a class of drugs known as neuroleptics, and the disorder they cause often is labeled by the rather cumbersome term *neuroleptic-induced tardive dyskinesia*. That two-word description tells it all. Tardive is derived from the word tardy, or late, and implies that the disease occurs late in the course of neuroleptic treatment, often after years of continuous treatment. Dyskinesia comes from two Greek words and merely means abnormal movements.

But what kind of movements, exactly? Chorea. The same brief, random, purposeless movements that are characteristic of Huntington's chorea. Hence its inclusion in the differential diagnosis of any adult who manifests chorea. Such is the nature of progress.

Tardive dyskinesia has become the bane of American psychiatrists. It is not rare. It occurs in 10 to 15 percent of psychotic patients treated with neuroleptics for years. In many of the patients the movements are mild, almost unnoticeable. In others, more a nuisance than a symptom, but in a small but significant number, the movements cause severe and often permanent disability. And the drugs the psychiatrists prescribe cause this disease. Without neuroleptics, there is no T.D. Causation is well understood. There is one basic risk factor for the development of T.D. and that is long-term exposure to neuroleptics under a doctor's orders. But without the neuroleptics, a patient might well remain overtly psychotic, requiring long-term, if not permanent, institutionalization. To treat or not to treat. Not to treat may mean years of psychosis. To treat may mean T.D. It's a risk. A calculated risk. Psychiatrists, as a result, find themselves between a rock and a hard place.

Most schizophrenics are treated with neuroleptics. Untreated psychosis is rarely a reasonable therapeutic choice. And some of them, as a result, develop abnormal movements that look just like those seen in Huntington's chorea. How, then, do physicians tell the two disorders apart? One clue, the key clue, is family history. Huntington's chorea is hereditary. Tardive dyskinesia is not.

Huntington delineated the prototype of a classic Mendelian dominant disorder, forty years before Mendel's work was published in any Western language. Obviously, Huntington's disease can occur without a family history. This can come about in one of two ways. One would be the spontaneous generation or mutation of the Huntington gene, said to occur perhaps once for every one or two million live births. The other results whenever the true biological father is someone other than the putative parent. This is known as adultery and is said to occur somewhat more frequently than one in a million live births. Exactly how much more frequently is unclear.

But when that occurs, the diagnosis of Huntington's disease cannot be easily made. To diagnose Huntington's, you need both a clinical picture consistent with Huntington's (psychiatric features and chorea) *and* a positive family history — an affected parent. Without the latter, one can be very suspicious but not definitely certain. And then nothing short of an autopsy helps. If a patient had chorea and psychosis and his parents lived beyond fifty without Huntington's, you can never be sure of the diagnosis prior to death. That individual could have any of a number of neurological or psychiatric disorders accompanied or complicated by chorea. And diagnosis of Huntington's cannot be made unless one is 100 percent certain. Not only because of the dire prognosis that follows, but primarily because of the implications for any offspring. Each child of a patient with a Huntington's faces the fifty-fifty prospect of developing the disease and being able to pass it on to his or her offspring. That is a burden that is far too heavy to be handed out lightly.

But what else could such a patient have? Our old friend tardive dyskinesia. A patient presents with a psychiatric disorder and is placed on neuroleptics. A year later, someone notices choreatic movements. Mild, brief, intermittent. Are they new? Or newly noticed?

What are they?

Chorea.

Why?

Is it tardive dyskinesia?

Or Huntington's following its natural course?

And how to tell which it is?

There are no tests for tardive dyskinesia.

And no tests for Huntington's chorea. A CT scan can give a clue, but not definitive proof.

A dilemma.

Tardive dyskinesia is what Mrs. Sarah Cook developed. Huntington's disease is what she didn't have. And the confusion of one for the other led to a lawsuit.

Sarah was in her early forties when her troubles began. She was married, with three teenage children. She was more than just unhappy with her lot. She felt worthless. Life was not worth living. Not at all. After weeks and months of tears and tantrums, she became frightened. Someone was plotting against her, poisoning her, trying to kill her. She needed more than simple outpatient management, so her psychiatrist admitted her to a psychiatric hospital. There all did not go well. Her depression did not respond to a trial with one standard antidepressant drug, so she was placed on a neuroleptic named Haldol, and her depression began to lift. In less than two months, she was able to return home.

Several months after her discharge, Mrs. Cook developed abnormal involuntary movements that resembled chorea. Her psychiatrist had never noticed them before. Were they T.D. or not? Had he caused them? Could she stay on her medicine? If she couldn't, would she become depressed again? What to do? He sent her to see a neurologist. After all, neurologists are the experts on abnormal movements. He could tell if she had T.D. If she did, they might have to change her medications and face the consequences. If she didn't, then the medications could be continued. The neurologist examined her. He watched her movements and made a diagnosis, not of T.D. but of Huntington's chorea. The family was told the diagnosis and the prognosis. And soon learned the genetic implications. They were all stunned, especially the oldest daughter, who was about to become engaged.

Their mother's future was bleak. Huntington's chorea is inexorably progressive.

Psychosis.

Dementia.

Chorea.

Falling.

Immobility.

Permanent institutionalization.

A slow and agonizing death, in some state hospital or other.

And each of her three children had a fifty-fifty chance of developing the same disease, with the same prognosis, which they could pass on to their children, if and when they had any. Not exactly the blessing they had hoped to pass on to the next generation.

They asked the neurologist if there was any way to tell which of them might have inherited the disease and which hadn't. That way they could decide about having children. No, he informed them, but a Dr. Klawans in Chicago was looking into the question.

They called me.

I told them that my research was all very preliminary, that I was not in a position to use that research for actual genetic counseling and, besides, they weren't eligible for the research or for any genetic counseling, for that matter.

Why not?

In order to be eligible for the research, I had to be certain of the diagnosis of Huntington's chorea. That meant that there had to be affected individuals in two consecutive generations (parents and grandparents, for instance). That would confirm the dominant inheritance of Huntington's. The same would be true if there had been pathologically proven disease in an affected parent. That meant an autopsy after their mother died.

But their mother was still alive, they told me. She was back home and, aside from the movements, she was doing well.

There was nothing I could offer them.

The next I heard about Mrs. Cook was four years later. Not from her children, but from her lawyer, Carl Samuels.

Mrs. Cook had gotten worse and worse. Each month the movements became more severe, more disabling. Each month they went back to the neurologist. Each month the neurologist shrugged his shoulders and reminded them that Huntington's chorea was a progressive disease. What could they expect? They did not need such reminders. They lived with that progression day in and day out. The neurologist increased the neuroleptics and the movements got worse. And as Mrs. Cook's movements became more pronounced, she became more and more depressed.

So each month they also took her to the psychiatrist, and each month he shrugged his shoulders and reminded them that Huntington's chorea was a progressive disease. What could they expect? They did not need such reminders. They lived with that progression day in and day out. And the psychiatrist further increased the neuroleptics.

And so it went for several years. By then the chorea, which had been so mild at first, was totally incapacitating. The family took Mrs. Cook to see a second neurologist. His name was Ben Appell. He took a history. He examined her. He asked about the family history. There was none. He told them that without a family history, he could not make a diagnosis of Huntington's chorea. Were they certain no one else in the family had ever had a similar illness?

Of that they were certain.

Then he could not make a positive diagnosis of Huntington's chorea.

Then what else could she have?

Tardive dyskinesia, he suggested.

What was that? they asked.

He told them.

They'd never heard of T.D.

Hadn't the psychiatrist warned them about the possibility of tardive dyskinesia?

No.

What should they do?

Stop the neuroleptic.

Why?

Tardive dyskinesia can be reversible. If the neuroleptics are stopped, the movements might get better. Especially if the medication is stopped as soon as the movements appear.

But she had had movements for several years already.

It was still worth a try.

They tried. The attempt was a total failure. If anything, the movements became more pronounced and so did her depression. Once again she became paranoid and suicidal and had to be re-admitted to the hospital.

The family consulted a lawyer. Their mother did not have Huntington's. She had T.D., a disease caused by her medicine. Shortly thereafter, a suit was filed.

Against whom? The lawyer, like most lawyers, wanted to sue everyone in sight. Anyone who participated in her medical care who should have known about T.D. and whose knowledge could have resulted in an action that might have changed her outcome. And I mean everyone.

The doctors.

The nurses.

The hospital.

The manufacturers of Haldol, the neuroleptic she had been treated with.

His theory of the case was rather simple. Everyone had screwed up. Starting with the psychiatrist, Dr. Wittgenstein. He had started her on Haldol. His deviations from the standard of care were almost too numerous to list, but list them he did. Wittgenstein should never have initiated treatment with Haldol. Haldol is not, after all, an antidepressant. It is an antipsychotic. It is used to treat schizophrenia, not depression. Had he never used Haldol, she would never have developed T.D. Furthermore, even if she had had schizophrenia and his use of Haldol had been appropriate, Wittgenstein had still deviated from appropriate medical care. Tardive dyskinesia was a well-known and serious risk of long-term Haldol therapy. He had not warned Mrs. Cook of the risk and had thereby abrogated her rights as a patient to accept or reject a treatment based on appropriate information. He had not recognized T.D. when it first appeared. And he had continued Haldol in the face of early, mild T.D., which had allowed the T.D. to become progressively more severe.

So much for Dr. Wittgenstein.

Next on his list was the neurologist, Charles Van Ness. He, too, had failed to make the correct diagnosis and had, in fact, made the wrong diagnosis of Huntington's chorea. This mistake had played a pivotal role in Mrs. Cook's being continually treated with ever higher doses of Haldol.

Other doctors were also involved. Internists who saw her in consultation at various times in her course. Other psychiatrists who saw her in the various hospitals where she was admitted from time to time. None of them suggested that she had T.D. nor did they act appropriately. None of them even raised a red flag or warned of the possibility of T.D.

Why were the hospitals liable?

They employed physicians (psychiatrists, residents) and psychiatric nurses who should have been able to diagnose T.D., and all of them failed to warn the patient or her family about the risk of T.D. resulting from long-term Haldol treatment.

And the manufacturer? For its failure to warn physicians and patients adequately about the risk of T.D.

In all, there were fifteen defendants — ten physicians, four hospitals, and one drug company. Six of the physicians, two of the hospitals, and the drug company all settled out of court. So that only four physicians and two hospitals were left when the case came to trial. I appeared as an expert for the plaintiff. As far as I was concerned, the major culprit was not the drug company or the psychiatrist, but the neurologist. True, the psychiatrist should not have used Haldol. Or at least not so quickly. His patient had been given a trial with only a single antidepressant. Others were available and should have been tried before resorting to Haldol. That is the standard of care. True, the psychiatrist should have warned the patient about the potential risk of developing T.D., but he had monitored the patient, and as soon as abnormal movements had appeared, he had sent her to see a neurologist. It was the neurologist's obligation to see those movements and realize that the patient could have T.D. and advise the psychiatrist of that fact. Then, if possible, Mrs. Cook should have been taken off Haldol and treated with true antidepressants. Had that been done, in all probability, the T.D. would have improved or at worst remained a mild disorder, all but inapparent. That did not happen. Van Ness made a diagnosis of Huntington's disease, a diagnosis he should never have made as a definitive diagnosis without a family history, and he never even considered T.D.

Where had he been over the last ten years?

Not in the library keeping up with the literature on T.D. It was as if he were still practicing medicine in the early sixties, and T.D. did not exist. But he wasn't, and it did exist.

As did his liability.

The jury gave Mrs. Cook over one million dollars. It was the first malpractice case in which T.D. resulted in a million-dollar verdict for the plaintiff.

It was not all that much money, considering the outcome. Mrs. Cook has severe contorting movements that she cannot control. There are no medicines that can help her. The standard ones we use, reserpine and tetrabenazine, tend to cause severe depression in susceptible individuals. And no one could be more susceptible than Mrs. Cook. So she remains severely disabled, a stage on which are played out a random succession of twists and jerks. Her tongue flys out of her mouth, her neck jerks to the side, her back arches, all but throwing her off her chair. And as she tries to catch herself, her head falls toward the floor.

That's her T.D.

It depresses her. How could it not? So as a result, the million dollars is being eaten away paying for her chronic inpatient care.

There is a constant refrain in medical circles that the awards that juries give to patients are far too high. So are the settlements that insurance companies reach with plaintiffs. Millions of dollars. And for what? Some abnormal movements. In a patient who was already disabled by depression. There is another refrain, equally loud and just as persistent. "Don't testify for plaintiffs. Don't get involved, even if the patient is a patient of yours and even if the plaintiff might have a valid complaint."

I hear these remarks over and over again from doctors, hospital administrators, deans. Even from medical students. They are almost always paired with complaints about the high cost of malpractice insurance and the need to practice defensive medicine. It's all but a continuous barrage. Often from people who are both friends and colleagues of mine. I always listen politely. Usually that's all I do. Arguing, I have discovered, does not help. It is like arguing religion. Belief in the right of a patient to have legal recourse for an injury resulting from malpractice is like belief in God. It is not a belief that can be inculcated by logical argument. Every time I am tempted to concede that my colleagues may have some degree of justification, I pull out a copy of Mrs. Cook's hospital bills.

The award was not sufficient.

SUIT TWO

Loose Lips Sink Ships

— World War II Slogan

There is one reliable way to differentiate dentists from physicians. The first time a dentist looks in your mouth, he shakes his head and tells you that all that dental work for which you spent so much money is of substandard quality and has to be replaced. Your previous dentist was, in short, incompetent. A new doctor takes your history, examines you, and no matter what he finds, smiles and tells you that your old doctor did everything just right. Perhaps not the way he would have done it, but don't worry, your previous doctor was an excellent physician.

— Richardson's Law

Donna Larson had never been a very happy woman. She had not had much schooling. She'd had to quit high school and go to work before she was sixteen. She got married a couple of years later to a man in his forties. The marriage didn't last very long. He drank a lot. That did not surprise her. She had met him at work, while she was working as a waitress in a bar. What did surprise her was that when he was drunk, he became abusive. She wasn't so much worried about herself. She could defend herself. But her baby, her baby: that was a far different matter. She walked out on him, taking the baby and what few other things she could carry.

Her timing was perfect. Less than two months later, while driving to church on Sunday morning and already drunk, he drove off a bridge and was killed. They had always driven to church together. Every Sunday morning, and he always drove. She felt very lucky to be alive.

Life went on.

She remarried less than two years later, to another man she met at work. She still had the same job, of course. She had more kids. She quit work and in time, her second husband began to drink more heavily. And when he got drunk, he, too, took out his anger on her, but only verbally. That was a plus of sorts.

The kids got older and went to school, so she went back to work.

Her last kid graduated from high school and moved out of the house, leaving her alone with her husband. Her unhappiness ripened into frank depression.

She felt worthless. Life just wasn't worth living. Finally, her oldest daughter took her to see a psychiatrist named Turley.

Dr. Turley talked to her and started her on a mild tranquilizer. He thought it would help. It didn't. Her symptoms escalated. Vague fear turned into terror. Suspicion became abject fear of all strangers. Her dislike for crowds evolved into an immobilizing inability to leave the house. The psychiatrist abandoned the mild tranquilizers. Instead, he tried antidepressants. Tofranil. Elavil. Nardil. Others too numerous to list. None of them helped her. Finally, he admitted her to the hospital. There he tried more antidepressants, in higher doses. She got no better. Something new was needed. Something different. He called in a neurologist to see her. The neurologist examined her and found no evidence of any neurological disease. The next day, she was placed on Prolixin. It, like Haldol, is a neuroleptic, an antipsychotic drug that is primarily used to treat schizophrenia.

The Prolixin did not help her. Nor did Haldol, which was tried next.

What was left?

There weren't too many options.

Finally, as a last resort, she was given a course of electroconvulsive therapy (ECT or EST — electroshock therapy — shock therapy, for short). But it, too, did not help. Her depression never abated. Her family was desperate. Her husband, especially, and his desperation and frustration quickly turned to anger. He became abusive to the nurses and the doctors. Finally, Dr. Turley suggested that the family might be happier if they sought a second opinion.

The husband agreed.

Mrs. Larson was transferred to a large psychiatric hospital. There it was noticed that she had abnormal involuntary movements. Choreatic movements! That meant that she had a neurological problem, but which one? What was her diagnosis? Did she have tardive dyskinesia? That was certainly a possibility. After all, she'd been on neuroleptics for six months, and that duration of continuous therapy was long enough to cause tardive dyskinesia.

Or did she have Huntington's chorea? There was no family history. So no one made that diagnosis. It was a possibility, but not much more than that.

Or did she have some other neurological disease? A neurologist named Alston saw her and studied her as thoroughly as he could, using the most sophisticated techniques, CT scans, NMRs, EEGs, blood tests. What have you. Nothing suggested any evidence of atrophy of the brain. Huntington's would, in all probability, show at least some degree of atrophy.

In the end, Alston reached no absolute conclusion. He couldn't be certain what disease Donna Larson had, but he did know what she could have and what that meant. She might have tardive dyskinesia and might therefore be better off if the neuroleptics were stopped. So he told her husband that she might have tardive dyskinesia. He became livid. That SOB of a psychiatrist had poisoned his wife. Turley, that bastard.

That was not the reaction Alston had anticipated. Far from it. He was not saying that the previous doctors had done Donna any harm. She had needed a trial of neuroleptics. Nothing else had helped. And if she had tardive dyskinesia and they stopped the neuroleptics, she might improve. And besides, he wasn't saying that she definitely had tardive dyskinesia.

"What else could she have?" the husband demanded to know.

It was possible that she could have Huntington's chorea.

"Huntington's chorea," the husband sputtered. "What's that?"

"A neurological disease."

"You mean she wasn't just crazy and didn't need all those medicines?"

"Not if she had Huntington's."

By now the husband was redder than a boiled lobster.

"Huntington's," he repeated.

"We can't be sure," the neurologist reminded him.

"That lousy SOB. He should have known what she had."

The concept that the doctor still didn't know precisely what his wife had eluded the husband entirely. The neurologist's efforts to influence Mr. Larson's rage were all unsuccessful.

Why hadn't Turley made the right diagnosis? He had worked with her for a year. Pills of all sorts, then ECT. And all those bills. Why the hell hadn't he known what she had?

The neurologist gave up. He was getting nowhere, and it was taking far too long not to get there.

Why didn't Turley make that diagnosis?

"Ask him," was the answer Alston gave to Mr. Larson.

"That SOB screwed up," was Larson's only reply. "He should have known she had Huntington's."

He'd give it one more shot. "She might well have tardive dyskinesia," he reminded the husband.

"What's tardive dyskinesia?"

Dr. Alston explained it again as carefully as he could.

Red became purple this time.

A side effect of her medication!

"Why the hell did he poison my wife?"

Alston gave up. "Ask him."

Mr. Larson did just that. The very next day. Over the telephone. He confronted Dr. Turley. "Why the hell did you hurt my wife?"

"Hurt your wife? I never did anything to hurt her. I tried everything I could to help her."

"You caused all her problems. I ought to sue your pants off."

"Sue?" The psychiatrist gulped.

"Damn right."

"But why? What did I do?"

"What didn't you do. For starters, you screwed up her brain with all those drugs."

"I what?"

"You gave my wife tardive dyskinesia," he said. "And never warned her."

Tardive dyskinesia.

The words added to Dr. Turley's fright. There had just been a successful million-dollar verdict for a patient who developed tardive dyskinesia. He didn't know any of the details, but that one, the million-dollar award, was all he needed to know.

Tardive dyskinesia.

He hadn't noticed any movements. The other doctors must have. They must have made the diagnosis. It was not a term that Larson could have come up with on his own.

"Did the other doctors tell you she had tardive dyskinesia?"

"Yep."

"Who?"

"A neurologist. A guy named Alston."

"What exactly did he tell you?"

"That she had tardive dyskinesia. And that you caused it."

Turley could see his professional life passing in front of him.

"And you never warned us."

He hadn't.

He was guilty.

That had been one of the issues in the million-dollar case. Failure to warn.

Damn.

"What did Alston tell you exactly?"

"That she might have tardive dyskinesia."

Might? Just might? He still had hope. "What else did he say?"

"That she could have Huntington's."

More than hope. There was a light at the end of the tunnel. And Huntington's was that light. "That's it. I thought she might. That must be it. Mrs. Larson must have Huntington's chorea."

"You didn't diagnose that."

"I know I didn't. I'm just a psychiatrist. I never diagnose Huntington's on my own. I leave that up to the neurologists. So I called in a neurologist. A Doctor Silvera. He saw her. He saw her in the hospital."

Silvera was not a name Larson had heard before. "Did Silvera say she had Huntington's?"

"No. Not at all. Just the opposite," Dr. Turley said. "Silvera told me that she didn't have any neurological disease. If he had told me that she had any neurological problem, I would have never given her those shock treatments. Patients with neurological disease can be made worse by shock therapy. That's why I made sure he saw her before I started the treatments. If only I'd known, I'd never have given her any shock treatments. That's what hurt her. Not me. If I'd only known. It's not my fault."

"That SOB," Mr. Larson concluded. "Silvera ruined my wife's life."

Dr. Turley was still worried, but it did seem that he was getting near the end of his tunnel.

"I'll sue that bastard Silvera, and you'll testify that it was because of him that you gave her those shock treatments that screwed up her brain."

The psychiatrist agreed. That way he was out of the tunnel.

And so the Larsons sued Dr. Ralph Silvera for not making a diagnosis of Huntington's chorea and thereby allowing Dr. Turley to give her the ECT, which "ruined" her.

They had the elements they needed for a successful malpractice suit:

Deviation: Failure to diagnosis Huntington's disease leading to,
Causation: Unwarranted treatment with ECT, which resulted in,
Damages: By ruining her.
Permanence: Forever.

All Larson needed was a lawyer who would accept his ludicrous theory of what had transpired. And then that lawyer had to find an expert to go along with that scenario. Neither was too hard to locate.

I acted as an expert, not for the Larsons, but on behalf of the defense. I was the expert witness for Dr. Ralph Silvera.

I was contacted by the lawyers retained by his insurance company. They had come across my name by running a library search for articles on Huntington's chorea and tardive dyskinesia. I was one of the few neurologists who had written articles on both subjects.

The lawyer, a man named Carl Tresh, called me and outlined his problem. I agreed to review the matter, and in due time a box of medical records and depositions arrived in my office. I read them all. In my mind, defending Ralph Silvera would be easy. He had not made a diagnosis of Huntington's chorea in Donna Larson because it had not been possible to make that diagnosis at the time he saw her. She had no chorea then, no abnormal movements, no signs of neurological disease at all. The fact was that no one had ever made a definite diagnosis of Huntington's chorea, not even a year later, when she had severe chorea. By the time of the trial, Mrs. Larson had been seen by two other recognized experts in movement disorders. Neither of them had made a diagnosis of Huntington's chorea. She did have depression and chorea, but there was no family history, and without that it was impossible to make a definitive diagnosis of Huntington's. You could be suspicious. I was. The doctors who treated her were. But no one was certain. If three years after chorea was present, the diagnosis remained unclear, the failure of Ralph Silvera to make that diagnosis was certainly not a deviation from the standard of care.

Not only was there no deviation, in my opinion, there was no causation.

True, the failure to make a diagnosis resulted in her receiving a series of ECT treatments, but for that to be causation, there had to be some harm. The ECT would have to have caused some damage. What actual harm had the ECT done?

As far as I could tell, the answer was none. The ECT, while it did no good, also did no harm to Mrs. Larson. During the time she received ECT, her clinical manifestations never changed. She got no better. She got no worse. She developed no new symptoms. None of her old symptoms got worse.

No harm meant no damages. And that, in turn, meant no causation. And of course, no permanence.

At trial, that became my testimony. Ralph Silvera had not committed malpractice. He had not made a diagnosis of Huntington's chorea when he examined her because no one could have. There was no family history. Even today, that diagnosis could not be made, and had not been made. To make the diagnosis would have been a deviation from the standard of care.

Why?

Because of the genetic nature of the disease and the burden it would cause her children.

Then I testified as to the lack of damages.

No deviation.

No damages.

No causation.

End of testimony.

On to the cross-examination.

The Larsons' lawyer, a man named Irwin Snider, tried to attack my knowledge of Huntington's chorea. After all, his expert had said that Silvera should have made the diagnosis. Anyone should have. Deviation. And the ECT caused memory loss. Damages. Causation. Permanency. The entire litany. I was at the time secretary-general of the World Federation of Neurology Research Group on Huntington's chorea. If there was anything on which I was an expert, it was Huntington's. I had published a dozen or more articles on Huntington's. I had written on the problem of early diagnosis and early detection of the disease. Their own expert had grudgingly admitted to my acknowledged expertise. He had no choice. In his deposition, he had said that I was an expert whose opinion he respected. That was before the defense named me as their expert. At trial, he either had to contradict himself or admit to my expertise.

The attack on my opinions per se and my expertise lasted less than twenty minutes. A couple of forays. Nothing more. Not even a real skirmish.

That did not end the cross-examination, however, far from it.

The inability to attack a man's credentials or opinions never stopped a street fighter, and Snider was a street fighter. Attack the man. Attack his motives. His credibility. Cast him as a hired gun. Jack Palance out to shoot Alan Ladd in the back and then murder

Van Heflin at the homestead. Cast him as a prostitute, a whore who is willing to do anything for money, even lie.

That was what the cross-examination evolved into. The forces of injured innocence against this combination of Judas Iscariot, Mary Magdalene, and Dillinger, all rolled up in one. After all, Dillinger, too, had come from Chicago.

Was I being paid for my opinions?

"No," I replied.

"You aren't being paid?"

"No. I didn't say that."

"So you are being paid for your opinions."

"No. I'm being paid for my time." That may be a rather subtle difference, but a real one, nonetheless. An expert is paid an hourly rate for his time, not his opinion. And he gets paid the same amount whether the side that retains him wins or loses.

Somehow lawyers believe the fact that experts are being paid degrades the experts in the eyes of the jury. I doubt that. They see the confrontation of a lawyer and an expert as the struggle of two hired professionals. And they are all damn sure that they are both being paid — especially the lawyer. That fact somehow escapes most lawyers. The simple truth is that both sides pay their experts, ergo, all experts are in some sense hired guns, whores. Snider pays his experts, but that, of course, is different. Why? I have no idea, nor does the average juror. Every lawyer who has asked me this question on cross-examination in front of the jury has lost his case. I have not always testified for winners. But as soon as I'm asked this question, I know my side has probably won.

Why? Is it a sign of a desperate last-ditch effort to discredit the opposition? Or a sign of a second-rate cross-examination? It could be either. Or both. Or, there may be some other explanation, but the observation remains. It's the sign of a lost cause.

Had I been in court before?

Yes.

"How often?"

"A dozen times or so."

"As an expert witness?"

"Yes." There I was whoring around.

"Over how many years?"

"Twelve years." I may be a whore, but I only whored once per year.

And always for the defense? Defending rich doctors from injured patients?

"No. It's about fifty-fifty . . ."

"So you'll testify for whoever pays you." A subtle jab. If I only testified for the defense, I was a part of some big conspiracy to deprive patients of their just compensation; I was prejudiced; I worked only for doctors. If I testified for both sides, I was a whore who went to the highest bidder. I had no convictions at all.

Are juries too stupid to see through that approach? I doubt it.

The defense lawyer objected.

The objection was sustained.

I complained that I hadn't finished my answer. The judge told me to continue. I explained that I reviewed cases for both sides and turned down more than I accepted, but I was willing to testify in any case in which I had a strong belief, whether that belief was on behalf of the plaintiff or the defense. And that turned out to be about fifty-fifty.

They were not getting very far in portraying me as Mary Magdalene or Dillinger.

What next?

Even I was surprised.

They attacked my credentials.

Whenever I am presented to the court as an expert witness, I supply two documents — a curriculum vitae, a biography of my professional training and accomplishments, and a bibliography, a list of all of my publications. My being accepted as an expert is, in part, based on those documents. If they were fraudulent, so was I. No one had ever challenged them before.

We went over them line by line. I shuddered. Not merely because they were long, but because I'm a horrid proofreader and I was sure there were some glaring errors.

And the lawyer found one. Publication number 127. One of the 331 papers I had published in the last twenty years.

Did I recognize the title?

Yes.

Had I written the paper?

Yes.

Where had I published it?

I looked at the bibliography before I answered. There is no way I can remember where all 331 papers were published. "*European Neurology*," I said.

"What year?"

I looked again. "1972," I answered.

He handed me a bound journal. It was *European Neurology* for 1972. Was my article in it?

I looked. It wasn't there.

"Well, Dr. Klawans?"

"No, it's not there," I conceded.

Why not? I had told them that was where it had been published. Or had I lied?

"Not really. I made a mistake. True."

"A mistake. For all we know, that article exists only in your imagination and you lied to pad your reputation."

"No, sir. I just happen to be a sloppy proofreader."

"But an honest man?"

"Yes, sir."

"At least that's what you would like us to believe. But, you know, I spent two entire days in the library looking for that article, and I never found it."

Cross-examination was over.

It was time for a recess, and there I was with egg on my face.

Things did not look good for our side. The only hope was to resurrect my reputation during redirect.

But how?

I knew a possible way out. I called my office. I keep copies of all my papers in numerical order. I got my secretary.

She pulled out the file.

Did she have a copy of number 127?

She did.

I asked her to FAX it to me.

Immediately.

She did.

Five minutes later I was back on the stand for redirect. The defense had one shot to clear up my reputation.

"Dr. Klawans," he began, "could you identify this document before me?"

"I can."

"What is it?"

"Number 127 from my CV."

"And where had it been published?"

"In *Confinia Neurologica*."

"How could you confuse *European Neurology* and *Confinia Neurologica?*"

"Easily. They are both published by the same publisher. In Switzerland, by a publisher named Karger. The two journals have the same editors. And very similar covers."

"So the article exists."

"Yes, sir."

"You didn't just invent it to pad your bibliography."

"Of course not."

"Why couldn't Mr. Snider find it in the medical library?"

"I suppose he's not very good at finding things he doesn't want to find."

Snider objected.

His objection was sustained. But he'd lost his street battle. And the case.

The game was over. My side had won. I should have felt the thrill of victory. I didn't. The game had become monotonous. Boring. I was tired of it. Worse, I was aggravated by it.

Malpractice cases should never revolve on such issues. They should be resolved by sober contemplation of the merits of the case.

Deviation.

Causation.

Damages.

Permanence.

The usual litany.

Not on jabs between lawyer and expert.

Perhaps some day they will be. But that day is not here yet.

SUIT THREE

The Negligent Dr. Klawans

I don't want a lawyer to tell me what I cannot do; I hire him
to tell me how to do what I want to do.

— J. Pierpont Morgan

Robin Lytle was schizophrenic. She still is. She had suffered three
episodes of acute paranoid schizophrenia before she was ever referred to me. The first had occurred when she was seventeen. She
was walking home from high school when she was visited by the
Fire of God. The Fire told her that she was the Queen of Chicago
and that within a week she would be living in the palace with the
King.

"Be ready," she was told. "Trust no one."

She knew what she had to do in order to get ready. She walked
into the nearest clothing store and walked out with four brand-new
dresses. Fancier dresses than she had ever owned. Strapless. With
sequins. By the time the police caught her, she had walked out of
other stores with lingerie, nightgowns, shoes, two coats, and I
can't remember what else. It would be difficult to classify what she
had done as shoplifting. She had made no attempt to sneak any of
the items out of the stores. She had just walked in, made her
selection, and taken them with her. When the police asked her her
name, she replied that she was Robin the First, the Queen of
Chicago.

The police wanted to know why had she taken the clothes.

God had told her to.

Why?

To be ready for the King.

And who was the King of Chicago?

She could not tell them his name. God had told her not to trust
anyone. She certainly couldn't trust them. They were arresting the
future Queen of Chicago, which is precisely what they did.

She was immediately sent to a psychiatric hospital. There she saw a Dr. William Taylor. He made a diagnosis of acute paranoid schizophrenia and placed her on an antipsychotic medication named Navane. Within two weeks she no longer said that she was the Queen of Chicago, and within three weeks she stopped receiving messages from the Fire of God. In a month, she was discharged. No criminal charges were pressed. All the clothing had been returned. The shop owners realized she was insane.

Robin returned to high school. And remained on her Navane. She made weekly visits to a psychiatrist. Not the one she saw in the hospital; Dr. Taylor took care only of inpatients. He referred her to a psychiatrist named Ron Johnson. Johnson talked to Robin each week, and he continued her on her medication. Mostly he listened to her and watched her. He listened to her in order to assess her thinking. Was there any evidence of paranoia? Any grandiosity? Schizophrenic thinking? And he watched her in order to monitor the possible side effects of her medicine. Were there any abnormal involuntary movements? Anything to suggest tardive dyskinesia? Week in and week out, the answers to both questions were negative.

The major question for Dr. Johnson was whether she needed to stay on her Navane. Had she just had a single episode of abnormal behavior which would not recur? An acute reaction of adolescence? Or was she truly schizophrenic? With a lifelong illness?

There was only one way to tell. Ron Johnson slowly tapered her off the medicine. At first Robin did well. Beautifully. She had never felt better. She was off all the medicine. She was happy. They decreased her visits to once every two weeks.

She stopped coming altogether.

Dr. Johnson called to ask her why.

She told him she wasn't sure she trusted him anymore.

He called her parents to warn them that she might be becoming paranoid again. But Robin had told her parents the reason why she couldn't trust Dr. Johnson anymore. He had asked her to lie down on the couch without her clothes on.

The father called Dr. Johnson and told him never to call again. If their little girl needed to see a psychiatrist, they'd find someone else.

Why?

If Johnson didn't know the answer to that, he felt sorry for him. Then Mr. Lytle told Dr. Johnson to get lost and stay lost. "Don't ever bother us again. Or Robin. Ever."

There was nothing else Dr. Johnson could do.

A week later Robin was arrested again. She was found walking down the hall at her high school stark naked. She was, she told the security guards, on the way to meet her husband, the King, for a trip to paradise and had to bathe naked in the school's pool in order to cleanse herself. She was dirty. She had to become clean. Pure. Virginal. A walk in the pool would make her clean again. And pure. And a virgin.

The police never got involved this time. The principal called the Lytles. They called Dr. Taylor. They trusted him. He'd never made their little girl take all her clothes off.

Dr. Taylor put her back into the hospital and back on the Navane. Within six weeks she was ready for discharge. She needed constant care and supervision. But by whom?

Dr. Ron Johnson, of course.

The Lytles adamantly refused to let Dr. Johnson treat Robin. Why?

It took Dr. Taylor almost an hour to get the answer. And another hour to convince the Lytles that Robin's accusation had been part of the same paranoid attack that had culminated in her taking off her clothes in school.

Taylor trusted Johnson. The Lytles trusted Taylor. So Robin once again became a patient of Ronald Johnson. This time she remained on Navane. After all, his question had been answered. It had not been a single isolated episode. She had now had two attacks of psychosis. She needed continuous treatment to prevent such recurrences.

So Johnson saw her and listened to her and watched her.

Once a week for three months.

Once every two weeks for three months.

Once a month.

She graduated from high school. Could she go away to college? Where?

The University of Michigan.

Of course. Johnson knew a very good psychiatrist there. A Dr.

Kern. Johnson sent Kern a letter. Robin would call him and set up an appointment as soon as registration was over and she had settled into her classes.

And she had to stay on her medication, Johnson reminded her. Of course. She knew that she couldn't stop her medication.

So off she went to the University of Michigan.

And off the Navane. She was an adult now. Not a high school kid. She knew what she needed. And she didn't need Navane. Besides, drugs weren't good for the baby.

Registration week went fine. She got the classes she wanted. And classes got off to a great start. She loved the dormitory. And her new friends. They didn't know about her past. They didn't judge her. She could trust them. Sort of. They didn't know who she really was, that she had to keep a secret until the Prince was born. It was her secret.

She liked everything. Except football. She couldn't understand why everybody else liked football.

After four weeks, she stopped going to class. She couldn't trust the professors. They could see right inside of her, and see the baby, and who she really was. And they knew who the father was.

Thank God, she had a single room. That way Dr. Johnson could visit her every night. And they could make love every night. All night long.

He was feeding the baby, he told her. His baby. But she knew it wasn't his baby. Her baby was the Prince. That was her secret. She couldn't even tell Dr. Johnson.

Kern called Johnson. That patient he had referred had never made an appointment.

Johnson called the Lytles.

Robin was fine.

Were they certain?

Yes, they talked to her every week.

She hadn't made an appointment to see Kern yet. She had to do that.

The Lytles agreed. They called her. Had she seen Dr. Kern? No.

Why not?

He was a friend of Dr. Johnson.

So?

Didn't they know what Dr. Johnson made her do?

No.

Terrible things. Dirty things. And now she was going to have a baby. And he kept bothering her.

"That son of a bitch," Mr. Lytle screamed. "I'll kill him. This will cost him his license."

He called Taylor. Taylor would know whom he should call to make sure that Ron Johnson didn't rape any of his other patients.

Taylor let Mr. Lytle vent his anger and then told him that his daughter had never been raped by Dr. Johnson. Taylor was confident that Johnson had never seduced her. Or been seduced by her. This was all part of Robin's paranoia. Remember the last time.

They did.

Johnson doubted that Robin was even pregnant.

What should they do?

Drive to Ann Arbor. See her. Talk to her. Take her to Dr. Kern.

That's what they did.

As soon as the Lytles saw her, they knew that she was pregnant. All it took was one glance and that was obvious.

Who was the father?

Dr. Johnson.

Was she certain?

"Dad, I was a pure, clean virgin before. Now I'm dirty. I'm . . ."

"That son of a bitch. I'll kill him."

"Don't. He must feed the baby."

The Lytles weren't sure what she meant by that. Child support? She said no more.

They took her to see an obstetrician, David Brown. He talked to Robin. How long had she been pregnant?

"Four weeks."

The way her dress looked, it had to be more than that.

Did she know who the father was?

Yes. Should she tell him the real truth, she wondered. He was her doctor. He would make sure her baby was born perfect. She had to tell him.

Yes, she knew.

Who?

"Ronald Reagan. The president."

He examined her and called in her parents.

She was not pregnant. She had strapped a pillow to her stomach. She couldn't be pregnant. She was a virgin.

"I'm still pure," she said. "I will give birth to the Prince and I'll still be pure."

Brown called Kern. Kern admitted her to the hospital and put her back on Navane. Four weeks later she was transferred back to Chicago and remained in the hospital there under Dr. Taylor's supervision for another four weeks. Then back to Dr. Johnson. Her outpatient care became an unalterable routine. Once every two weeks she went to his office and he listened to her and watched her very carefully.

Six months later he noticed something. She was smacking her lips. Not often, but more than before. More than normal. And twitching her nose. And sticking out her tongue.

Abnormal movements! Were they the first signs of tardive dyskinesia caused by her Navane?

What to do?

Send her to the expert.

So she came to see me. Johnson had been right. She did have abnormal involuntary movements. A whole lot of them.

Lip smacking.

Tongue protrusion.

Jaw thrusting.

Nose twitching.

Eye closure.

Not often. Not severe. But enough to be abnormal. And there was no other cause. She had tardive dyskinesia as a result of the longterm treatment with Navane.

I called Johnson and confirmed his worst fears.

What should he do?

If possible, get her off all antipsychotic medications.

Impossible.

Why?

She had gone off twice before and become psychotic both times, and each time it had taken her longer to recover. Next time, she might not recover. Ever.

Then keep her on the lowest possible dose, I suggested.

That he was already doing.

Discuss it with her and her family so that they all understand the options. If she were to stop the medicines, the movements would probably get better, but her psychosis might recur. If she stayed on, the opposite could happen — increased movements, permanent movements, but less chance of psychosis.

He did that.

Everyone agreed the movements were the lesser of the two evils.

I saw her again six months later. She was still on Navane and the movements were still there. They were no worse and no better. Just there. Mild. Not enough to bother her.

That was the last time I saw her as a patient.

Two years later, as I was escorting a patient from my office through the waiting room in order to reach one of the examining rooms, a man stopped me. He was in his forties, potbellied, in an old checkered suit with a bright sport shirt and a hat. He looked as if he hadn't shaved in two days. I wouldn't try to guess when he had last showered.

"You Doctor Klay-wan-is?" he asked.

"Klawans," I corrected him. "What can I do for you?"

"Take dis, Doc," he said, handing me some paper. "You been served."

"Served?"

"Yep. I'm a deputy."

He was a deputy sheriff and I had been served. I was being sued. By Robin Lytle. *Lytle v. Johnson, Klawans, et al.*

I finished examining my patient and called Ron Johnson.

"You, too?" he replied to my initial greeting. He then brought me up to date on Robin Lytle.

She had continued seeing him for about six months, then she had met a guy. He was into health foods. And vitamins. Huge doses of vitamins. Megavitamins.

And no chemicals.

Robin at first went halfway. Health food and megavitamins, but she stayed on Navane, too.

Then her boyfriend suggested she see a megavitamin specialist. She did. The "specialist" told her to take even more vitamins.

Robin stayed on the Navane, but she stopped seeing Dr. Johnson.

She and her boyfriend got an apartment together. He threw out the Navane. Her movements got worse. He hated them.

Johnson had poisoned her, so had Klawans.

At first Robin knew that wasn't true. But her boyfriend was adamant. She had been poisoned.

The megavitamin specialist agreed. His name was Griffen. Archibald Griffen. He was a psychologist. He was the only one she could trust. Not even her boyfriend. They broke up. She moved out. And moved in with Griffen. He prescribed more vitamins, bigger doses.

Now she knew the truth. Johnson and Klawans had poisoned her. She went to see a lawyer, an Anthony Branoff.

And now we had been sued.

I read the papers. The charges were that both Ronald Johnson and I had been negligent in our roles as "psychiatrists." We had made the wrong diagnosis. She had a vitamin deficiency, not schizophrenia. We had given her an unreasonably dangerous drug and caused permanent harm to her and her two children, who were both severely retarded.

What children?

I was aghast.

I called the hospital's lawyer. Since I am an employee of the hospital, he is also my lawyer in matters such as this. I told him about the lawsuit.

"I'm not a psychiatrist," I complained.

"So what?"

"I never diagnosed her as being schizophrenic. I never treated her for schizophrenia. Whatever damage she had from the neuroleptics was there before I ever saw her."

"So what?"

"They lied in the lawsuit."

"So they'll amend it later." Suing for something that hadn't happened, it seems, is within the rules.

I called a friend, David Kramer. Dave's a lawyer who specializes in malpractice. I told him the entire story. "What can I do?" I asked.

"Nothing."

"But I am not now nor never have been a psychiatrist."

"I know."

"I never treated her for schizophrenia."

"I know."

"Can't I sue her?"

"Probably not."

"Can I sue Branoff?"

"For what?"

"Filing a frivolous suit? He never bothered to review my records or Johnson's. She's crazy, told Branoff a crazy story, and he sued me."

"No. She has a right to a day in court. And a right to representation. She can sue him for negligence. But you can't."

"That's one hell of a way to run a railroad."

"It's the law. And don't forget, we lawyers write the laws. And lawyers need all the protection we can get."

"That's some system."

There was very little more to do. It was obvious what had really happened. Robin, influenced by her boyfriend and Dr. Griffen, had gone off Navane. And her paranoid psychosis had returned. And her paranoia had been fed and directed toward me and Ron Johnson.

And all we could do would be to try to defend ourselves.

Over time the complaint became modified.

I was no longer charged with being a "psychiatrist" who had been negligent. I became a negligent neurologist.

Then one "child" disappeared.

Then the other.

Why?

No one ever said.

Then she gave her deposition. She was frankly psychotic. She talked about her brain-damaged children. She had never been pregnant. Her parents took her straight to William Taylor. Taylor hospitalized her and put her back on Navane.

She stayed in the hospital for five months. She then came under the care of a Dr. Leach. Leach saw her every week. To listen to her and watch her.

He noticed some abnormal movements. Mild at first, but then more definite.

Did she have tardive dyskinesia?

And if so, what should he do?

He told her she had to see in expert on movement disorders. Who?

Dr. Harold Klawans.

So she called my office to make an appointment.

What should I do? I had no legal obligation to see her. She had terminated my care of her by failing to return in over three years. I had no obligation to initiate care again, especially not of a patient who had sworn out an affidavit saying that she believed that my prior treatment had been negligent.

I called David Kramer.

He called Branoff. I would be more than willing to see Robin if she dropped the suit, with prejudice, meaning that she could not refile it.

"Never," he said. He would send her to some other neurologist, which is just what he did. But the other neurologist told her and her parents that she should see me. I was the expert.

Her parents went with her to see Branoff.

"No. Never." She should go back to see Dr. Taylor. She did. He told Robin that she should see me.

Back to Branoff. He finally relented. But only when Mr. Lytle hinted that he might sue Branoff if his little girl got any worse. And "hinted," I'm sure, was too weak a term for what Mr. Lytle said. The case was dropped. Robin made an appointment to see me. On the way to my office, God visited her again. She was stopped by the police. She was walking down the middle of the street, screaming that President Reagan had abandoned their child.

The last I heard, she was still in the hospital.

And back on Navane, with mild, but ever-present abnormal movements from her tardive dyskinesias.

EPILOGUE

The Crab

Not to know the events which happened before one was born, that is to remain always a boy.

— Marcus Tullius Cicero
(106–43 B.C.)

Elizabeth Berry used to be the "in-house" counsel for Smith Kline Beckman. She managed many of their legal problems, including malpractice/product liability suits. When I first met her, SKB was still SKF (Smith, Kline and French); it had not yet purchased Beckman and broadened its base from pharmaceuticals to include medical instruments and laboratories. SKF introduced Thorazine, the first successful antipsychotic drug, to the U.S. market in the early fifties. SKF had not developed Thorazine. That had been done in France, where it was called Largactil. SKF had purchased the exclusive license to sell Largactil in the United States and had given it the name Thorazine.

As the first pharmaceutical company to introduce a neuroleptic to the United States, it was only fitting that SKF be one of the first manufacturers to be named as a defendant in a lawsuit based upon the occurrence of neuroleptic-induced tardive dyskinesia. The plaintiffs in such suits frequently name both the treating physician (for malpractice) and the manufacturer (for product liability). As an outsider, I often felt that the inclusion of the manufacturer was usually based not so much on true liability as it was on two other factors. The first of these is the deep-pocket theory of law. This theory teaches that the plaintiff must always sue the person with the most money, that is, the deepest pocket. Since the defending physician may have only a limited amount of insurance, there may well be more money available for quick settlement if the drug company is included. Almost all malpractice suits are disposed of before trial. Some are dropped. Many are settled. In any such settlement, the most that is ever asked of a defendant is the limit of his or her insurance policy. In such discussions, it is always assumed that the resources of the manufacturer are unlimited. The second factor only comes into operation if the case goes to trial. Most malpractice cases that go to jury are found in favor of the defendant. To the jury, it is a question of person versus person, injured plaintiff versus caring physician. The human factors often cancel each other out. But that balance can be shifted. Sue the drug company and it becomes injured patient versus faceless corporate entity. And that's no contest.

The issue in all such suits, as far as the manufacturer's involvement is concerned, is always the same — the failure to adequately warn the unsuspecting patient and the treating physician. As an expert on tardive dyskinesia, I have often been consulted by drug companies on this issue. Smith, Kline and French was one of the first companies to contact me in this regard. It was Elizabeth Berry who contacted me. She managed all their malpractice cases. She did not actually defend them. She did not personally take depositions or go to court. The company hired local counsels who lived and practiced within the jurisdiction in which the suit was filed to do that. But she arranged for the appropriate expert witnesses. That's the downside risk for the plaintiff in including the drug company as a defendant, one which many lawyers overlook. If you sue the drug company, you are suing a defendant with expertise in defending such cases. And that expertise often includes both a thorough understanding of the medical and scientific issues that few other lawyers have and a knowledge of who the real experts are and what their opinions are likely to be.

It was late on Thursday evening when Elizabeth Berry called me about a case in which SKF was a defendant. By then we knew each other fairly well. I had already acted as an expert for SKF in a couple of cases. There was another case she wanted to discuss with me. SKF, of course, was "one of the defendants." The issue, of course, was T.D.

"Failure to warn?" I suggested.

"What else?" she replied.

"When?"

"Nineteen seventy-five."

"Your warnings were adequate then."

"I know," she said.

The case was in a rural jurisdiction in Vermont. It was already in trial.

Why had I not been contacted sooner?

The local counsel wanted to use local experts. He felt that the average Vermont juror didn't trust outsiders.

So why now?

Things were not going well.

Did the plaintiff really have T.D.? I inquired. That was always the first line of defense. Much better than an opinion that the warning included by SKF in the package insert was adequate. After all, if the patient did not have T.D., but some other non-drug-related neurological problem, then Thorazine could not be blamed for anything.

"Absolutely."

"Why are you that certain?"

"She's been seen at National Institutes of Health. They diagnosed her as having T.D. She's even been published in a couple of their studies."

"Who at NIH?" I asked.

She told me.

I recognized the name. He was a psychiatrist and a recognized authority on T.D. I'm always skeptical of a neurological diagnosis made by a psychiatrist, but this psychiatrist had been studying T.D. for years. "She's got T.D.," I concurred.

Would I review the records?

I would. Over the weekend. They should send them out by express mail.

They arrived Saturday morning. I spent most of the weekend reading them. Medical records, depositions, trial testimony. Even the published papers in which the plaintiff was one of the subjects.

Smith, Kline and French was in trouble.

The plaintiff had severe T.D. She was only thirty-three. That meant she had a life expectancy of more than forty years. She had had T.D. for five years and was still totally disabled by it, and, more probably than not, she would be totally disabled for life. Thirty years of total disability. Assume she made $20,000 per year. A reasonable assumption, since she was a college graduate. And if one corrected for inflation of 5 percent per year, that represented over a million dollars in lost income alone.

Add to that pain and suffering, and it was easy to see that SKF was in trouble. Start with a million dollars in lost income, and add a helpless victim with grotesque, contorting gyrations of her body. So what if the big, impersonal drug company brought in some out-of-town, hired gun to say that their warning had been adequate.

No matter that the physician should never have put her on Thorazine in the first place. She had psychiatric disease, but she was not schizophrenic and she had never been psychotic. She had hysteria and severe anxiety, neither of which is an indication for the use of Thorazine. Other medications are both safer and more effective. The physician, like SKF, had been in trouble, but his insurance company had already thrown in the towel and given the plaintiff his entire policy ($200,000). The doctor's sole defense had been that he didn't realize this could happen.

Why not?

Smith, Kline and French had not warned him. They were in big, big trouble. Million-dollar trouble.

There was only one more piece of evidence to review. A videotape of the patient done at NIH to document her response in one of their drug studies. She had been put on an experimental antipsychotic and antianxiety drug that did not cause T.D. and that some thought might even help T.D. She had responded dramatically, but the drug had to be stopped because it caused liver problems in some other patients. The tape was VHS. I had Beta. I'd review it Monday morning at the hospital. It was just an exercise. I already knew she had T.D.

On Monday, I got into the hospital at eight, made rounds until ten, and then took the tape down to the education resource center to watch it.

A title came on the screen — Subject Nine, pretreatment. Then came the patient. She appeared pleasant enough standing there. No facial movements. No jerks, no twists, no nothing. Just a wan smile.

What T.D., I wondered to myself.

Then it happened. Like a bolt out of the blue. Her head tossed back, her knees bent. She swayed backwards, her arms extended behind her. Then she was on all fours, her feet planted just where they had been and her arms straight back, hands flat on the floor with her eyes gazing at the ceiling. Her back arched like a bridge. Her head kept moving back. Her arms bent until she rested not on her hands, but on her head. A three-point stance, her feet and her head bridged by her body. Her arms now lifted off the floor and extended laterally from her body.

"This," a voice said, "is the beginning of her dyskinetic spell."

Then she began to move counterclockwise. Like some giant crab. She rotated around her head, first moving her left foot to the left and then her right in the same direction, balancing herself by shifting her arms.

"This is a full-blown movement," the voice continued. "This usually lasts for ten or fifteen minutes at a time."

I turned off the tape. SKF was in no trouble at all. She did not have T.D. She had one of the more notorious of all patterns of abnormal movements ever described by a neurologist. It had been described in the 1880s by Charcot, the first professor of neurology, as the classic, typical expression of hysterical epilepsy — epilepticlike attacks due not to brain disease, but to hysteria. Charcot was not only the premier neurologist of the world, he was also the preeminent authority on hysteria. Freud had traveled to Paris to study with him, as had countless others.

Charcot had described precisely what I had just witnessed, not as a neurological problem, but as a manifestation of psychiatric disease. Everyone had accepted that to be true, even Charcot's most bitter enemies. What had caused the controversy was whether this set of movements was common or not. Charcot said it was common, the typical manifestation of hystero-epilepsy. He saw it every day of the week, in dozens of patients. He even gave it a name, "arc de cercle." One of his students, Gilles de la Tourette, made a drawing of one of Charcot's patients. That drawing was a classic of late-nineteenth-century clinical illustration.

Others said it was not just rare, it was very rare, perhaps even nonexistent, and certainly not a typical movement of hysteria. They said it was a secondary manifestation of hysteria, caused by the influence of Charcot himself. All his patients were on one ward. If a patient had a hysterical attack of the type Charcot had been studying, that patient was given immediate and prolonged attention by the professor himself. All other attacks got less attention. Soon, the patients all had the same type of attacks.

Charcot refuted the criticism. The battle was joined. Today, we know that both sides were right. Such attacks are hysterical. But they are rare. They became common only in the artificial setting of Charcot's ward of hysterics. A small chapter in the history of nineteenth-century neurology, a cul-de-sac, a bit of arcane knowledge known well by a fair number of neurologists, but few, if any, psychiatrists. And the patient had been diagnosed as having T.D. by a psychiatrist.

I dug up my copy of the Gilles de la Tourette drawing. It could be superimposed on the posture of the plaintiff. She did not have T.D. She did not have any neurological disease at all. Her movements were psychiatric in origin, and everyone agreed she had psychiatric disease. That was why she had been put on Thorazine in the first place. No wonder she got better during the trial on an antianxiety drug.

I called Liz Berry.

"Good news," I said.

"We settled," she said.

"Why?"

"The psychiatrist from NIH had shown his tape. It had made the jury cringe. They felt they had no choice."

"You should have called me sooner," I said.

"Why?"

"She doesn't have T.D."

"Doesn't have T.D.?" Liz echoed softly.

I explained what the tape had shown, but it was too late. The case had been settled. When had they settled? Just that morning. The expert had shown the tape to the jury at about the same time I had been looking at it.

"Next time," I said, "call me sooner."

"I will."

"And send a Beta tape."

"Why?"

"I can watch it at home and call back a day sooner."

"Better yet, I'll buy you a VHS." And she did.

CHAPTER FOURTEEN

Crazy Like a Fox

In Jerusalem I asked
the ancient Hebrew poets to forgive you,
and what would Walt Whitman have said
and Thomas Jefferson?

— Paul Potts

In the beer and espresso bars they talked
of Ezra Pound, excusing the silences of an old man
saying there is so little time between
the parquet floors of an institution
and the boredom of the final box.

Why, Paul, if that ticking distance between
was merely a journey long enough
to walk the circumference of a Belsen
Walt Whitman would have been eloquent,
and Thomas Jefferson would have cursed.

— Dannie Abse, 1958
"After the Release of Ezra Pound"

In recent years, I have found myself increasingly drawn to the works of physician-writers and not just those whose writing had been so well accepted that they deserted the practice of medicine, like Conan Doyle and Chekov. I have become more interested in those who continued to juggle both endeavors, such as William Carlos Williams. So it was with great anticipation that I entered the world of the poetry of Dannie Abse. I had been rummaging through the Rush Medical College bookstore when I came across his *Collected Poems*. As always, I started with the back cover,

which told me that this was the first collected edition of his works
and was drawn from five books of poetry that had received out-
standing reviews. I was about to replace the book on the shelf
when I read the last line of the cover blurb. It told me that Abse
was Welsh, a fact that did not impress me, that he was married,
that he had three children, and that he lived in London, where he
continued to practice medicine. A British William Carlos Williams.

I immediately began to read through the book, turning the pages
to find any poems with titles that caught my mind and reading
those in their entirety. Those I read, I liked. They were well crafted
and communicated at least some of their meaning in a direct way.
Then I got to page sixty-four, and the title jumped out at me,
"After the Release of Ezra Pound."

"How," I asked myself, "could any self-respecting poet write a
poem about that anti-Semitic, fascist son of a bitch? They should
have lined the treasonous bastard up after the war and shot him."

I was tempted to put the book back, not where I'd gotten it, but
hidden at the back of some obscure rack, to collect its well-
deserved share of dust and grime. Ezra Pound, indeed!

Instead, I read the poem. It opened with a quotation from another poet, asking the ancient Hebrews to forgive Pound his sins.
I became more incensed. It was a veritable conspiracy of poets to
somehow resurrect one of their own. Let the rest of the world be
led into the gas chambers, but Ezra Pound was a poet and, as such,
above any guilt. He had to be forgiven.

"The sons of bitches!" I said aloud, no longer limiting my dis-
gust to just Abse or Pound.

I read on.

And came to the last two stanzas, which condemned not only
Pound, but all of his apologists, more eloquently and more pow-
erfully than I ever could. This was not forgiveness. This was vengeance and truth.

I bought the book and ordered six more copies to give to friends
of mine. It was a very good day.

I had first become aware of the existence of Ezra Pound during my
first year as an undergraduate at the University of Michigan. That

was 1955, and the twin shadows of the House Un-American Activities Committee and McCarthyism still hung over the country. But things were beginning to change. Pete Seeger was coming to Ann Arbor to give a concert. Pete was one of the messiahs of folk music, but he had been blacklisted as a dangerous subversive. Seeger had actually made a record of the songs of the Lincoln Brigade, that group of Americans who had gone to Spain to fight against Franco and the fascists. What could be more subversive!

I went to the concert. Not as a political act, but because I liked listening to Pete Seeger. The concert, of course, attracted all the left-wingers, would-be bohemians, and artists — the great unwashed, as my father referred to them. After the concert, one of them circulated a petition, one that no self-respecting American could refuse to sign. It requested the release from some mental institution of somebody named Ezra Pound. I had never heard of Ezra Pound. Before I could ask who he was, the bearer of the petition educated me.

"Our government stinks. Pound is the greatest poet since Shakespeare. Greater. And they keep him in a mental prison. Why? Because he has seen through their hypocrisy."

"What hypocrisy?" I asked.

I got a very sullen look.

"Which particular one?" I added, clarifying my original question.

"The international conspiracy to control money, for one."

I stopped listening. I had to. It sounded too much like the beginning of the great lie: *Mein Kampf* revisited. I did not sign the petition, but the next afternoon I spent several hours in the library trying to learn about "the greatest poet since Shakespeare."

Pound, I learned, had been born in 1885 in Harley, Idaho, and was generally considered to be a poet's poet. Perhaps that explained why I'd never heard of him, never read a single line of his poetry, and could not find his name in the catalog of courses given at the University of Michigan. In 1907, after receiving an M.A. from the University of Pennsylvania, he took a job as professor of romance languages at Wabash College in Crawfordsville, Indiana. He had already begun writing poetry and living a bohemian lifestyle. Neither went over too well at a Presbyterian college in Crawfordsville, Indiana, in 1907. He was fired for "suspicion of moral turpitude."

He immediately set off for Europe, where moral turpitude was better tolerated. And there he stayed for the next forty years, except for short sojourns in the U.S. He wrote numerous volumes of poetry and criticism and had a profound influence on much twentieth-century writing in English. He was among the first to recognize and review the poetry of Robert Frost and D. H. Lawrence. He persuaded the already famous and respected William Butler Yeats to adopt a leaner style of writing, the style on which his fame now rests. He collaborated with James Joyce, overseeing the publication of both *Portrait of the Artist as a Young Man* and *Ulysses*. He edited and contributed to many of the early works of T. S. Eliot, including "The Wasteland." He helped Hemingway launch his literary career. Perhaps he wasn't the greatest poet since Shakespeare, but he may well have been the greatest editor since the unknown editors of the Old Testament.

In 1924, Pound moved to Italy and became increasingly interested in economic theory. He came to believe that the world needed monetary reform, that a total misunderstanding of money and banking by governments was the cause of most, if not all, wars and depressions. He became an admirer and supporter of Mussolini.

I began to shudder.

During the Second World War, he made hundreds of propaganda broadcasts on Rome radio in which he openly condemned the U.S. war effort and urged U.S. troops to mutiny. He went so far as to proclaim that the U.S. government was controlled by Jewish bankers, as was the world economy. The great lie.

He was, I learned, an anti-Semitic son of a bitch. A fascist. A Nazi. And he was guilty of treason. Why had he not been shot? Lord Haw-Haw, the British citizen who made similar broadcasts for Hitler, had been executed. Why not Ezra Pound? After all, even I knew that treason at the time of war was a capital offense. So why had he gotten off?

In 1945, Pound had been arrested by U.S. troops in Italy, and after spending six months in a camp for military prisoners near

Pisa, he was sent to the U.S. to be tried for treason. However, there was never any trial. He was declared "mentally unfit to stand trial" and placed in St. Elizabeth's Hospital for the Criminally Insane in Washington, D.C., where he still resided.

BULL! I said to myself.

Several days later, the petition passer ran into me on campus. He had noticed that I had not signed the petition. He pulled out a pen.

I shook my head.

"Why not? You were at the Seeger concert. You're not one of them?"

"You can't have it both ways."

"Both ways?"

"Is Pound insane?" I asked.

"Of course not. The government is incarcerating him for his political views."

"If he's not insane, he should be shot for treason."

"But he wasn't guilty of treason. He was insane."

"You can't have it both ways," I repeated. "He can't be innocent because he's crazy and a martyr because he's not crazy."

"He's a poet. The greatest poet since Shakespeare. You can't judge him by ordinary standards."

"He's a treasonous, anti-Semitic SOB. He should be shot."

"He's above such judgment."

"No one is above such judgment."

It was not until I was working on the manuscript of this book that I gave much more serious thought to Ezra Pound. As I was writing about the Dan White case, the parallels to Ezra Pound began to reverberate in my head. Were not the issues the same? Had not both men avoided the appropriate punishment because of supposedly altered mental/psychiatric *capabilities?*

Perhaps. But there were questions that had to be answered first. Many questions:

Had Pound been guilty of treason?

Had Pound been insane?

Had he been treated and later improved?

What had happened to him? All I knew was that he had died in Italy, as a free man. And that he had never spent a day of his life in prison.

Had psychiatrists really collaborated to protect him? And if so, why? Because he was a genius?

Pound remained in St. Elizabeth's for twelve years. During those years, he did not receive active therapy for any psychosis. He was never diagnosed as being psychotic. In the early fifties, neuroleptics were introduced and given to millions of schizophrenics and psychotic patients in mental hospitals throughout the United States, but not to Ezra Pound. Shades of Dan White. During his stay, he continued to write his own poetry, and to translate ancient Chinese poetry. He even translated a play of Sophocles, *The Women of Trachis*. And he received visitors regularly. He had regular private liaisons with both his wife and numerous mistresses. He had his own specially designated and protected private quarters in which he held literary seminars, meeting regularly with such colleagues as T. S. Eliot, William Carlos Williams, Archibald MacLeish, e.e. cummings, Robert Frost, and Margaret Hamilton. A regular literary salon, at government expense, for a man charged with treason.

But was he so crazy that he could not stand trial? That he could not cooperate in his own defense? That the government had no choice?

I doubt it. He never underwent psychotherapy. He never underwent any formal treatment. No formal diagnosis was ever made.

In his twelve and a half years at St. Elizabeth's he was examined by forty psychiatrists. According to Dr. Harold Stevens, one of his psychiatrists in the hospital, "The consensus held that he was of sound mind, could collaborate with counsel, and demonstrated no psychosis."

But had he been guilty of treason?

A few excerpts from his recorded broadcasts answered that question. Pound started making these in 1941. They were all recorded in Rome. Every month he would travel from his home in Rapallo to Rome, presumably on the railroads that ran on time, and record a group of seven-minute talks that were initially broadcast ten times a month to North America and, as the war evolved, to U.S. soldiers in the field.

On the February 19, 1942, broadcast, he complained, "that any Jew in the White House should send American kids to die for the private interests of the scum of the English earth . . . and the still lower dregs of the Levantine."

In April of '42, he said, "Don't start a pogrom. That is, not an old-style killing of small Jews. That system is no good, whatever. Of course, if some man had a stroke of genius, and could start a pogrom up at the top, I repeat . . . if some man had a stroke of genius, and could start a pogrom up at the top, there might be something to say for it. But on the whole, legal measures are preferable. The sixty kikes who started this war might be sent to St. Helena, as a measure of world prophylaxis, and some hyper-kikes of non-Jewish kikes along with them.

"For the United States to be making war on Italy and on Europe is just plain damn nonsense, and every native-born American of American stock knows that it is plain downright damn nonsense. And for this state of things Franklin Roosevelt is more than any other man responsible."

In June, he added: "You are not going to win this war. None of our best minds ever thought you could win it. You have never had a chance in this war."

And in 1943, he continued on his merry way: "Just which of you is free from Jewish influence? Just which political and business groups are free from Jewish influence, from Jew control? Who holds the mortgage, who is the dominating director? Just which Jew has . . . nominated which assemblyman indebted to whom? And which one is indebted to Jewry or dependent on credit which he cannot get without the connivance of Jewry?

"What are you doing in the war at all? What are you doing in Africa? Who amongst you has the nerve or the sense to do something that would be conducive to getting you out of it before you are mortgaged up to the neck and over it? Every day of war is a dead as well as a death day. More death, more future servitude, less and less of American liberty of any variety."

If this was not treason, I don't know what was. Lord Haw-Haw had said nothing worse and he had been tried and executed, but not Ezra Pound. Why not?

In June 1943, Pound was indicted in absentia by a Washington, D.C., grand jury. According to the indictment, Pound "knowingly, intentionally, willfully, and unlawfully, feloniously, traitorously, and treasonably did adhere to the enemies of the United States . . . giving to said enemies of the United States aid and comfort within the United States and elsewhere."

Pound continued to make his broadcasts, but the fortunes of war were changing. An Allied victory became inevitable. The Italians resigned from the war. German troops took over Italy. Still the Allies advanced. Rome fell. Pound took to the hills. There he was faced with one of two prospects. He could remain in the hills and chance being recognized and captured by Italian partisans and shot without benefit of a trial, or he could surrender to the U.S. Army and take his chances with the due process of U.S. justice. Ezra Pound was no fool. He decided to surrender to the Americans. The first soldier to whom he presented himself had no idea who he was or what he was talking about and refused to take him prisoner. Such is fame. Finally, Pound located an officer who knew who he was and was willing to arrest him.

At first, Pound was kept in an outdoor cagelike structure, then he was transferred to the U.S. military prison outside of Pisa, where he was allowed use of a typewriter and produced his *Pisan Cantos.* After six months, he was brought back to the U.S. to stand trial.

At his initial hearing, Pound argued his own case. He believed that his supposedly treasonous behavior was protected by the constitutional guarantee of freedom of speech. According to newspaper reports, his argument was eloquent and logical, though not persuasive enough; he was held for trial.

He then obtained a lawyer, Julien Cornell, and with the lawyer, a new strategy. Cornell, in his book *Trial of Ezra Pound,* described their first meeting and the new strategy:

"I discussed with him the possibility of pleading insanity as a defense and he had no objection. In fact, he told me the idea had already occurred to him."

Even Pound must have realized that it was not a good time to be tried for treason. Several Nazi collaborators, including Pierre Laval in France, and the eponymous Vidkun Quisling in Norway, had been tried, found guilty, and executed. Lord Haw-Haw had also been convicted and was awaiting execution in England.

The decision to claim insanity raised two separate potential ploys. The first could be to claim that he was not sane enough to cooperate in his own defense. The second could have been to plead that his treasonous acts had been carried out at a time when he, because of insanity, could not prevent them. The latter could only be addressed if Pound was sane enough to stand trial. At that time, the McNaughton rule applied. Under this legal principle, Cornell would have had to prove that Pound did not know the difference between right and wrong when he committed his alleged acts of treason. That would have meant proving a severe degree of psychiatric disorder, either continuously or off and on for the better part of three years. No easy task.

The issue became whether Pound was sane enough to stand trial. If he wasn't, when had he become insane? On that Pound was clear. These two weeks in the "cage" had driven him insane. Those two weeks had done it. Few, if any, of the millions of Jews and others in far worse conditions in Nazi concentration camps were driven insane, but somehow this had been sufficient to push Ezra Pound over the edge.

Again the parallel to Dan White is striking. Had Ezra Pound eaten Twinkies in that cage?

Ezra Pound was not tried for treason. A panel of four psychiatrists examined him and together came up with the unanimous opinion that Pound, because of insanity, could not collaborate in his own defense.

No collaboration.

No defense.

No trial.

Off to Saint Elizabeth's. Not because he had been crazy during the war when he made his treasonous broadcasts and advocated genocide, but because he was too insane at the time of the hearing to stand trial. But was he really insane?

There was a major dissenting opinion that Pound was sane. No one who held that opinion was called upon to testify. Three U.S. Army psychiatrists had examined Pound in Pisa. All three felt that he was sane. None of them was ever asked to testify. Nor were any of the large group of psychiatrists at St. Elizabeth's ever called as witnesses.

Dr. Harold Stevens, a neurologist and psychiatrist, spent many hours interviewing Pound during Pound's years in St. Elizabeth's and never detected any evidence of psychosis. One of his progress notes (dated March 31, 1946) epitomizes his observations:

> This patient has been interviewed on several occasions throughout the month, most of the sessions beginning with a complaint of fatigue which Mr. Pound accompanied by histrionic gestures designed to emphasize his alleged state of complete exhaustion. As the interviews proceeded, he ignored his obviously feigned infirmities, becomes quite animated in his conversation, bangs the desk, jumps up, raises his voice, becomes flushed and displays evidence of energy, the interview often lasting an hour. At times his speech is fragmentary, although telegraphic in style, resembling the cryptic letters he writes. In fact, his present style of speech and writing resembles his poems and other artistic productions. He is apparently a true Symbolist, who compresses a large volume of words and concepts into a brief expression. It seems that often a distinct remark is meaningful to him, but the complete meaning is lost on others. His language is often esoteric, but does not represent condensation in a schizophrenic sense. Often when asked to amplify an obscure remark, he will reply that his ideographic processes move rapidly but are not distorted or obtunded. Disbelief was not conveyed to him, but when he was queried about his selection, "Faces in the Metro," he confirmed the above impression. He states that his oversimplified work was a result of repeated and arduous deleting, striking, and reorganizing, over a very long poem, finally reducing to one esoteric sentence, which, to the interviewer, conveys very little of the original meaning. This extreme economy of style still characterizes his speech and writing, and

while he may be obscure he is never disconnected or irrelevant.

In frequent discourses with him, he is unable to answer some questions because of an alleged partial amnesia which he states developed during his confinement in the "cage" in Italy. However, when he is questioned about his earlier poetic works, for example, "Concava Vallia," his memory appears perfectly intact as he expatiates at great length on this and on other neutral subjects. But when queried about his scurrilous and anti-Semitic broadcasts in Italy, which the interviewer has reviewed, he protests that his memory fails him. On one occasion when he was asked if he wishes to stand trial, he effected an elaborate caricature of fatigue and the interview had to be terminated. He is in complete contact with his surroundings, and apparently appreciated his predicament. Intellectual processes are well integrated, and his genius is quite apparent. No abnormal mental content is elicitable, and there has been no evidence of hallucinations, delusions, ideas of reference, or ideas of alien control. His views on economics, and especially on money, are unorthodox, but logical and coherent.

The prosecution employed three psychiatrists as expert witnesses. All three examined Ezra Pound. They were Dr. Winfred Overholser, superintendent of St. Elizabeth's Hospital and soon to become president of the American Psychiatric Association; Dr. Marion R. King, director of the Mental Health Division of the U.S. Public Health Service; and Dr. Joseph L. Gilbert, head of the psychiatric section of Gallinger Municipal Hospital in Washington, D.C. The defense employed only one expert, Dr. Wendell Muncie of Johns Hopkins University. The three government witnesses agreed that Pound's psychiatric state was such that he was not capable of collaborating in his own defense. Muncie initially considered Ezra Pound to be of sound mind, but was then persuaded by the other three psychiatrists to join in an expression of unanimity, declaring Pound incapable of collaborating with his counsel. Dr. Overholser was the main witness at the trial and the apparent choreographer of the event. He gave his opinion and that was that. After all, he was an expert for the government. One could not expect the prosecution to give him a hard time. They picked him. If they hadn't liked his opinion, there were a lot of psychiatrists with opposite opinions whom they could have subpoenaed to testify. Needless to say, the defense accepted his testimony. The jury deliberated a grand total of three minutes and they found Ezra Pound of unsound mind and unable to cooperate with counsel. Pound was then remanded to St. Elizabeth's Hospital. As it would be thirty years later in the Dan White case, it was not the defense that carried the day, but the prosecution.

But why? After all, Pound had been guilty of treason.

The answer is unclear. There are two separate issues here, the role of the prosecution and the role of the psychiatrists. Ever since Freud, many psychiatrists have viewed themselves more as humanists than scientists. Many apparently felt that a writer of Pound's accomplishments and contributions to literature and to the development of so many other great writers should not be judged by the same standard as mere mortals. Was this the basis of Overholser's behavior? E. Fuller Torrey, a psychiatrist who worked at St. Elizabeth's after Pound's discharge and made a thorough study of the Pound affair, interviewed Dr. Carlos Dalmau, a colleague of Overholser. Dalmau told Torrey that Overholser considered Pound to be a great poet and that although Pound had made "mistakes," he should not have to face the risk of execution. Another psychiatrist who was at St. Elizabeth's at that time, Dr. Jerome Kavka, put it this way, "Ezra Pound was an exceptional poet and so he deserved exceptional treatment." It has also been suggested that Overholser's major motivation may have been to avoid a public circus in which St. Elizabeth's and its staff might end up occupying all three rings. For years, Overholser had tried to protect the public image of psychiatry by urging private conciliation of legal issues, avoiding the public disagreements among opposing expert psychiatric witnesses in the open courtroom. How embarrassing would it have been if the divided members of the St. Elizabeth's staff appeared on both sides of the issue? He was not the first psychiatrist to take this position. Dr. William A. White, Dr. Overholser's predecessor as superintendent of St. Elizabeth's Hospital and himself a renowned forensic psychiatrist, had played a similar role in the Leopold-Loeb murder case. White had tried to get the experts for the prosecution and the defense to confer together and to have the three families each of which had lost a son come together and reach a constructive conclusion, thus avoiding a courtroom battle that could embarrass the field of psychiatry.

But what about the prosecution? What explains their acquiescence?

To that I have no ready answer. Did they, too, wish to avoid the circus? Did Pound have friends in high places? Or as Fuller Torrey suggested, were they afraid that their case was too weak? That argument leaves me unimpressed.

In 1949, Pound was named the recipient of the Bollingen Prize for Poetry for his *Pisan Cantos,* poems written while in Pisa, after the two weeks in the cage that had caused his diminished capacity. This award for achievement in American Poetry was to be awarded by the Library of Congress. It was established in 1948 with money given by Paul Mellon. Mellon was an admirer of Carl Jung, the Swiss-born psychoanalyst, and the award was named after the town in Switzerland where Jung spent his summers.

The announcement of the award caused a scandal. Pound was still under indictment for treason. A congressional committee demanded that the Library of Congress dissociate itself from the award, which was transferred to the library of Yale University.

A rather quaint story. Innocent in a way. But not as innocent as it seems. The award had been given to Pound in an attempt to force his release from St. Elizabeth's. Archibald MacLeish, his friend, and a frequent visitor to St. Elizabeth's, was head of the Library of Congress and organized the conspiracy.

It backfired. The incongruity of a poet who was too demented to stand trial and at the same time capable of writing poems that could win such a lofty honor was not overlooked by writers, columnists, psychiatrists, and much of the general public. Pound had to stay in St. Elizabeth's. He might have had enough friends and supporters to save him from facing trial, but not enough to set him free.

In 1958, a second hearing was held. Pound was once again declared to be permanently insane, incurable. This man who had received no drugs, despite twelve years of incarceration, more than half of which followed the introduction of neuroleptic drugs for the treatment of psychosis, was insane and would remain so. According to whom? Our old friend Winfred Overholser, ex-president of the American Psychiatric Association and still super-intendent of St. Elizabeth's. In his sworn affidavit, Overholser declared that Pound was still "suffering from a paranoid state which has rendered him and now renders him unfit to advise prop-erly with counsel or to participate intelligently and reasonably in his own defense and that he was and is and has continuously been insane and mentally unfit for trial." In essence, "he is permanently and incurably insane." Pound was, however, not dangerous, so he was released into the custody of his wife with the understanding that he would leave the U.S. And they did, traveling back to Italy with his mistress. In Italy, he greeted most visitors with a Nazi salute.

Pound died in 1972, a free man. He had returned to the U.S. only once, to receive an honorary degree from Hamilton College. The trustees of that institution should have known better.

In 1946, a writer named Albert Deutsch had asked a simple question: "Is it possible that psychiatry can be used as a cloak to protect an accused traitor from possible punishment?"

Unfortunately, the answer is "Yes."

But not just in 1946, and not just accused traitors.

How does this differ from the more recent Russian misuse of psychiatry which the World Federation of Psychiatry, spearheaded by a later president of the American Psychiatric Association, con-demned?

Not as much as we would like to believe.

AUTHOR'S NOTE

> I am seldom interested in what he [Pound] says, but only in the way he says it.
>
> — T. S. Eliot

There is still a tendency in most literary articles to overlook Pound's treason and his anti-Semitism, as there has been to ignore T. S. Eliot's anti-Semitism. Shakespeare had it all wrong. It is not the good that men do that is oft buried with them, but the evil. Both are wrongs that should be corrected. It is just as reprehensible to underestimate Pound's pivotal role of editing Joyce and Eliot as it is to overlook his "mistakes"; they were not mere social indiscretions. Only revisionist historians uninterested in the truth would ignore what was for many years the major theme of Pound's life. Unfortunately, many of his biographers have chosen to ignore reality. Fuller Torrey does not. His book *The Roots of Treason* (McGraw-Hill, New York, 1984) and his brief article "The Protection of Ezra Pound," *Psychology Today* (57–61, 1981) are both recommended and have been used as major sources for this study.

As I was starting to put together my thoughts for this essay, I recalled that Harold Stevens, a noted neurologist from Washington, D.C., whom I knew as a professional colleague, had at one time been at St. Elizabeth's. I called Harold to ask him if he knew anything about the Ezra Pound affair.

"That anti-Semitic SOB," he replied. "We should have shot him, the treasonous bastard."

"What about his insanity . . ."

"What insanity?" he interrupted me. "Pound was never crazy. Everybody protected him. It was reprehensible."

"I like a man who understates his views," I said.

Harold then told me that he had been one of Pound's doctors in St. Elizabeth's and that he had put together an article for a proposed history of St. Elizabeth's Hospital, entitled "Ezra Pound and the Sheltering Arms of St. Elizabeth's." He then sent me a copy of his paper. Some of his observations are quoted directly from this article. Many of the points made in this article were originally emphasized by Dr. Stevens.

I still read physician/writers whenever possible, but ever since I started serious study of the Pound affair, I have been unable to read William Carlos Williams. Somehow, my view of the universality of his humanity has been diminished. Perhaps I am too cynical.

"How," I asked a friend of mine, "knowing what Pound had said, could he remain a friend of Pound's, even if they had been friends ever since they were undergraduates together?"

"There are," he replied, "some issues over which reasonable men can agree to disagree.

"Genocide is not one of those issues."

CHAPTER FIFTEEN

Where There's Smoke

Smoking is a shocking thing—blowing smoke out of our
mouths into other people's mouths, eyes, and noses, and having the same thing done to us.

— Samuel Johnson
(1709–1784)

I saw Sandra Sharp for the first time on December 7, 1977. The
Chicago Tribune that day had, for the thirty-sixth time, reprinted
pictures of the destruction wrought by the Japanese surprise attack
on Pearl Harbor, a practice which they have regrettably allowed to
lapse. She had come to see me because she wanted the answer to a
single, simple question: should she have an operation or not? She
had been told that she should, but she had been told that by the
surgeon who wanted to perform the operation. She wanted another opinion. She knew that brain surgery could be quite dangerous and she already had enough problems. She had gotten my
name from someone she knew. He had said I was a very good
neurologist. I had treated his father.

"Who?" I asked, always interested in knowing which of my old
patients and their families referred other patients to me.

She couldn't remember the name of her friend or his father.

That did not surprise me. It had taken almost twenty minutes to
tease out why she had actually come to see me, why she had
wanted to see any neurologist. Her neurological problem was obvious. The particular question she needed answered was not. Sandra Sharp had aphasia. Aphasia is the term neurologists use to
describe difficulties with the symbolic use of language. Language,
not words. Not sounds. It's not a problem with the mechanical,
muscular production of sounds or words. It's a problem in under-

standing and producing meaningful speech or language. She was twenty-seven years old and she was aphasic. Her aphasia was painfully apparent to both her and to me. She primarily suffered from what is sometimes called nominal aphasia, a word-finding difficulty, an inability to come up with the right name, the correct noun, the wanted linguistic symbol.

Why? What had happened to her?

It was a story she had told many times before, to several other doctors. She knew all the facts. She even had them straight in her head. It was just that sometimes they came out wrong.

She smiled. The expression on her face was somewhere between a smile and a blush. Her aphasia still embarrassed her. And her smile was not normal. It was asymmetric. Not bad enough that the casual observer would notice it, but any neurologist would. We are not casual observers. The right side of her face did not move as well as the left side. But that asymmetry involved only the lower part of her face. That was a sign of disease of the left side of her brain. The left hemisphere, the area where the control of speech is located.

The facts were as follows:

She was twenty-seven years old. And, I observed, a very good-looking twenty-seven-year-old, with long red hair, pleasant features, and a striking figure. I know I'm supposed to be a neutral observer, but I am an observer, nonetheless.

She had been on birth control pills for over ten years, ever since her senior year in high school, just after her sixteenth birthday. She smoked a pack and a half of cigarettes a day and had for more than ten years. To epidemiologists and others interested in the cumulative effects of cigarette smoking, that represented fifteen pack-years. That was sufficient to be a significant factor in her health. Age sixteen was to me a very early time in life to start either smoking or birth control pills. That had been the early sixties. The age of revolution.

Otherwise, she had been healthy. No high blood pressure. No heart disease. A clean bill of health.

She was a college graduate. She had been a teacher, then changed professions. All of this took over twenty minutes to relate.

"I became a legal . . ." she smiled. It was her same asymmetric smile.

"A legal what?" I asked.

Her smile changed into a look of asymmetric puzzlement. "A legal . . . you know what. A whatchamacallit. Letters, typing . . . You have a medical one."

"A secretary," I suggested.

"Yes," she agreed, "a legal one. You know what."

I did.

Then, less than two months earlier, that had all changed. She remembered getting out of bed at three in the morning. Someone was at the door. She opened the door. It was a friend of hers. She had known him for a year. He said, "Hi."

She said nothing. She tried to, but no words came out. Not his name. In fact, she couldn't even remember his name. She could not even say, "Hi."

She smiled.

He looked at her strangely. She certainly hadn't said anything wrong. And he had seen her in a nightgown before. Hell, he had seen her in a heck of a lot less. She smiled again.

His look changed to one of concern.

Was there something wrong with her smile?

He asked how she was.

She smiled again.

"Are you okay?"

She nodded.

"Can I come in?"

She nodded again. She hadn't seen him in months. But they were friends. They'd been lovers. Good friends. Good lovers.

He came in. He put his arm around her. His face pressed down onto her. He kissed her. She felt his tongue enter her mouth. She wanted to respond. But her tongue wouldn't do what she wanted it to.

He thought she was not responding.

She wanted to.

Didn't he understand?

Then her right hand went numb. Her right arm felt very heavy. Her right leg felt weak. Very weak. It crumpled under her, and she crashed to the floor.

Her friend, the one whose name she could still not recall, picked her up and carried her to her bedroom and laid her down on her bed.

Not now, she thought. Didn't he realize that something was wrong?

He started to lift up her nightgown.

Stop! she thought.

She wanted to tell him to stop.

She had to.

Her mouth fell open.

Wordless.

Mute.

She was naked.

She had to stop him.

She tried to scream.

To shout.

"Fuck it all," she said.

"Don't worry," he said. "I'm going to dress you so that I can take you to the hospital."

She had given me a perfect history of the sudden involvement of classic expressive or Broca's aphasia. In that type of aphasia, there is a marked loss in the ability to express language, but understanding is relatively well preserved. It is named Broca's aphasia after the nineteenth-century French surgeon and anthropologist Paul Broca, who first demonstrated its relationship to a specific region of the left hemisphere. Patients with a Broca's aphasia often lose the ability to direct all tongue movements. Sandra had. And they frequently develop weakness of the right side of the body. She had manifested that, too. But expletive speech, emotional speech, and swearing, which come from the right half of the brain, are often preserved. These had remained intact in Sandra.

"Fuck it all," she had replied.

Obviously her speech had improved somewhat, but it was still far from normal.

Once she got to the hospital, she was admitted and seen in consultation by a neurologist. He confirmed that she was aphasic and had right-sided weakness. Sandra already knew that much, although, at the time, she didn't know what the word "aphasia" really meant. He also told her that she had had a stroke on the left half of her brain.

A stroke. Why? She didn't ask the question; she merely gave him a puzzled look. She thought that she was too young to have a stroke. After all, she was only twenty-seven. Strokes were for old people. Not her. Oh God! "Shit," she said.

The right-sided weakness cleared up over the next three or four days. The aphasia resolved far more slowly.

The doctors told her they wanted to do "a . . . special . . . ray of some sort."

"An angiogram," I suggested.

"That's the special one."

That might tell them why she had had the stroke.

She wanted to know that.

They did the special test. She had brought a copy of it with her. I looked at it. The doctors had told her that one of her thinga-mabobs was blocked up. Whatever blood was getting to the left hemisphere was coming from the supply route that normally sup-plied only the right hemisphere. The X rays showed that her left internal carotid artery was totally occluded.

I stopped her. Did she really understand all that?

She looked at me.

A smile.

Puzzlement.

Both uneven.

"Yes," she said. "I maybe do. I think. Sort of . . . Damn!"

I took the time to explain it to her. There are four main arteries that supply blood to the brain, two in the back called the vertebral arteries, and two in the front, the carotids. Each carotid has two divisions, the external, which goes to the face and scalp, and the internal, which goes to the brain. The left internal carotid supplies blood to the left hemisphere, but before it does that, there is a circle of blood vessels at the base of the brain, the Circle of Willis, where the arteries all meet, a sort of traffic junction.

"Like one of those things in England," she said, "a whatcha-macallit."

"Yes, a roundabout."

Her left internal carotid was blocked, so whatever blood her left hemisphere was getting was coming from other blood vessels.

"Through the whatchamacallit."

"Correct."

She understood.

The neurologist called in a neurosurgeon to see her. The neurosurgeon told her that she needed a bypass operation. This "simple" procedure would shunt blood from her left external carotid artery which normally supplied blood to the scalp to the internal carotid above the level of the block. A bypass. That would increase the blood supply to the left half of her brain.

"More speech?" she had asked him, in her typically telegraphic way.

"No," he replied.

"Why?"

"It will keep you from getting another stroke."

"Why did I stroke?"

The stroke, the neurologist explained, was from the birth control pills. The combination of birth control pills and her smoking. She should stop both, especially the smoking. Didn't she know that smoking was bad for her health? She should stop smoking. And have a bypass. These were what they recommended.

She didn't really understand why she needed the surgery. She'd had her stroke and she would stop smoking.

They said she needed it. Trust them, they were doctors.

But it was a doctor who had given her the birth control pills. Why should she trust doctors? And brain surgery wasn't ever simple. That much she knew.

She said no.

They recommended that she get a second opinion.

From whom?

Another neurosurgeon.

She decided to do just that.

They told her whom to see.

She followed their advice.

Neurosurgeon number two advised her to have the operation. It would save her from ever having another stroke. If she wanted, he'd do it himself. He had more experience with that type of bypass surgery than any other surgeon in Chicago.

She didn't trust him either, so she ended up in my office. I, at least, wouldn't try to operate on her, would I?

No. No. I didn't do any surgery at all. And certainly not any bypass operations.

What was my opinion?

She had had a stroke, I began, going step by step. The stroke was related to her long history of birth control pills plus heavy smoking. Fifteen pack years.

What should she do?

No more birth control pills.

What else?

No more smoking. And she should probably be on medications that might make such strokes less likely to recur.

What medicine?

"Aspirin, Persantine."

Would they help?

Perhaps. But they wouldn't hurt. The major factor was to decrease her risk for stroke by stopping the smoking and the birth control pills. There were other methods.

She laughed. Her laugh was completely even. No asymmetry. "Abstention for one."

She laughed again. "I haven't . . . you know . . ."

"Had sex."

"No," she laughed, "in so long. Thank you."

"You're welcome," I replied.

Then we got back to business. She wanted to know about the operation.

I wouldn't recommend it, I told her.

Why not?

That was the key question. The bypass procedure was all the rage at the time. It was a fairly new operation. Surgeons had been doing them for only a couple of years. Vascular surgeons had been doing carotid artery surgery for decades. Those operations are performed directly on the diseased carotid arteries themselves in an attempt to remove the diseased part of the artery and restore normal blood flow. The type of operation that had been recommended to Sandra was far different. She had a completely blocked carotid artery. Operating on her neck would not change anything. What the surgeon wanted to do was to open up her skull and connect a branch of the artery that normally went to her scalp to a branch of the artery that went to her brain. The latter, because of the blocked carotid in her neck, was not getting sufficient blood. The hope was that after the operation the blood from the external branch would supply more blood to the internal branch and thereby to her brain.

Unfortunately there were too many unanswered questions. No one had ever proven that the operation either improved recovery from a single stroke or prevented the occurrence of a second stroke in the future. It might, but then again it might not. And it had been done mostly in older patients who had different causes for their strokes.

As far as I knew, no one had ever even claimed that it prevented strokes in young women whose strokes had been caused by the combination of being on birth control pills and smoking. The notion was, I thought, preposterous. She needed to be off birth control pills.

She was.

And to stop smoking.

She'd try.

Sandra became my patient. I saw her every three months, mostly for reassurance. Eventually I got her to stop smoking. I sent her to a speech therapist. Over the next year, her aphasia improved even more, but her speech never returned to normal. She would never teach again. Or be a legal secretary.

After six months, she went back to work. First she tried working as a waitress. She couldn't keep the orders straight. But she needed to work. She moved up to hat-check girl. That was too frustrating. People expected her to respond to them. To their jokes. She couldn't follow jokes, especially if they included double meanings.

She became a clerk in a florist shop. It was the perfect job. She watered the plants. She arranged them. She even talked to them. They couldn't tell that she was aphasic. Then came Mother's Day.

She had to sell, to listen to customers, to talk to them. That she could not do, but she could add and subtract just fine. And she could run the cash register. That she could do anywhere, if that was her only responsibility. She went back to the restaurant. It was too fancy a place. She needed to do more than add and subtract. What she needed was some coffee shop or deli.

A coffee shop it was. She ran the cash register at a take-out coffee shop downtown. No words. Just numbers. And an occasional smile.

Slowly but surely her speech improved.

She tried more adventurous jobs.

Hat-check girl.

Waitress.

Clerk in a city office. Filing. Filling out a few forms. It was not as good as being a legal secretary, but better than being a hat-check girl.

There she ran into a young lawyer from the firm where she had been working when she had had her stroke. He asked her what had happened. She told him. He sent her to see a malpractice lawyer. The lawyer thought she had a great case. It included both product liability and medical malpractice. Two for the price of one. He would sue both the drug company and the doctor. The drug company because they manufactured a dangerous drug that had caused her to have a stroke. And her OB-GYN doctor because she had given her the dangerous drug that had caused her to have a stroke.

How much was he talking about?

He made a few quick calculations. Her present income was $11,000 per year. Before her strokes, she had made $23,000 per year. That was $12,000 per year for forty years. Almost half a million in lost wages alone. Two million, he guessed.

That sounded good to her. She could use two million dollars. She didn't like working as a clerk for the City of Chicago that much.

Minus his percentage, he reminded her.

And how much was that?

Thirty-three percent.

"Six hundred and sixty-seven thousand out of two million," she said. "That leaves me with one million, three hundred thirty-three thousand." After all, her math skills were intact.

It still sounded good to her.

What did they need to get started?

Experts, her lawyer said. Did she have a doctor who was an expert in neurology?

She did. Me. So in due time, I was asked to be one of her expert witnesses. Not for deviation from the standard of care. I'm not an OB-GYN. I can't testify as to the standard of care of OBs. I was to be the expert on the other issues. Diagnosis, causation, damages, permanence.

Diagnosis: Sandra Sharp had had a stroke. Her stroke resulted from an occlusion of her left internal carotid artery. The stroke had caused right-sided weakness and aphasia.

Causation: The stroke had been caused by taking birth control pills while smoking a pack and a half of cigarettes each day.

Damage: She had an aphasia that still markedly limited her speech.

Permanence: She would never get any better than she was.

The lawyer felt that their case was almost in place. All that was needed was testimony as to the deviation from standard of care on the part of her physician and as to a failure on the part of the manufacturer to warn the physician and the patient. Both would have to come from expert witnesses other than me.

These turned out to be far from trivial problems. They were the essence of the entire case. Without such negligence on the part of the physician who gave her the birth control and/or on the part of the company that manufactured the birth control pills, such issues as causation, damages and permanence would all be meaningless. They become irrelevant. Negligence was everything, for without proving it, she couldn't win the case.

There had been no failure to warn on the part of the pharmaceutical manufacturer. None at all. At one time, there had been. Medical science became aware of a relationship between birth con-

trol pills and strokes several years before the manufacturers put
adequate warnings of that danger in their package inserts. That had
been in the early seventies. And there had been successful lawsuits.
Young women on birth control pills who had strokes had sued and
won big settlements. Millions of dollars. But by 1977, the manufacturer's warning was clear. Birth control pills increased the risk
of a stroke, especially in heavy smokers. It was there in black and
white in the *Physicians' Desk Reference* which was sent to all physicians, and it was also in the package insert given out to each
patient with each month's supply of pills. The warning was there.
And it was adequate. It had been given to Sandra each and every
month. If she chose to ignore it or disregard it, or not even read it,
that was not the manufacturer's fault. You can lead a horse to
water, but you can't make him drink. That may not be the exact
legal principle, but that's how the law works.

The manufacturer was out of the case. That left the obstetrician.
Had she warned Sandra?

Yes. But Sandra didn't remember the warning.

The doctor, however, did. And she had recorded it in her
records. And she testified to that in her deposition. Her name was
Parnell. She was in her early seventies.

"I told Sandra that if she took the pill and continued to smoke,
she would have a stroke."

"Did she ever tell you that she had stopped smoking?" Sandra's
lawyer asked Dr. Parnell.

"No."

"And yet you went ahead and gave her the pill, even though you
thought it would cause her to have a stroke?"

"Yes."

"Why did you do that?"

"Because if I didn't, someone would have. I tried to get her to
use some other method of birth control. But she wouldn't. Dia-
phragms were too inconvenient. And condoms were out of the
question."

The lawyer had continued to question her about willfully giving
a harmful medication, but she didn't sway. She had done it knowing that if she didn't, someone else would.

The lawyer was pleased by Parnell's testimony. He was certain that he had her. She had admitted that she had given Sandra the pills knowing that she would have a stroke. That was just what he needed. She had willfully given her patient a harmful form of treatment. That was against the Hippocratic Oath, which told physicians that their first duty was to do no harm.

He was already counting the money.

The defense took my deposition. I talked about causation. I talked about damages. I talked about permanence. But I didn't talk about standard of care.

Had I read Dr. Parnell's deposition?

I had.

What did I think about what she'd done? Did I have any opinions?

Yes, I did.

What were they?

That she'd done the most that could have been expected of her. Dr. Parnell had knowingly given a drug that might cause a stroke, *but* she had warned her patient and she had been right. If she hadn't done it, some other OB-GYN or internist or GP would have. In 1977 that was still the standard of care.

Five years later it wasn't, but then it was.

Sandra's lawyer could see his case disappearing. "The Hippocratic Oath," he asked me. "You do believe in the Hippocratic Oath, don't you?"

"Of course not."

"You don't?"

"No. I don't believe in an oath to the god Apollo. And that's how it begins. 'I swear by the god Apollo . . .' "

Going . . . going . . . gone.

I still see Sandra once every three months. She doesn't smoke. She doesn't take birth control pills. She has her partners use condoms. She got started before they became popular.

Now thirty-nine, she still works as a clerk for the City of Chicago. She still has long red hair and a striking figure. And she has found happiness.

She is still aphasic, with significant nominal aphasia, but she has a guru. She has become a devotee of some Indian swami and she chants syllables in Hindi. She has no idea what they mean. But neither does anyone else who chants with her.

She chants away on an equal footing with everyone else.

Peace.

Serenity.

Nirvana.

Whatchamacallit.

AUTHOR'S NOTE

Why do birth control pills cause strokes? Or more precisely, increase the risk of developing a stroke? Probably by increasing the tendency of the platelets in the blood to stick together (platelet stickiness) and thereby sludge together and result in a thrombosis.

Why does smoking further increase this risk? Once again, the exact answer is not known. Perhaps by causing a further increase in platelet stickiness and thereby an increased tendency toward thrombosis. Perhaps an increased tendency of blood vessels to contract and thereby be more likely to become completely blocked by a small thrombosis.

But whatever the mechanism, the observation remains. It's an unhealthy combination.

Back when this case was going on, I didn't believe that external carotid-internal carotid bypass operations helped patients. I had recommended that Sandra not have the operation. The fact is that I never recommended a single one for any patient. But by the early eighties, everyone was doing them. The EC-IC bypass had become one of the country's top ten operations. Right up there with hernias and gall bladder surgery.

Why were they being done?

I was never certain.

Did they help?

As far as I was concerned, there was no proof they did.

Finally, the National Institutes of Health sponsored a cooperative study of some three thousand patients. The first definitive study. Its conclusion was that EC-IC bypasses were of no value.

The insurance companies stopped paying for them, so the surgeons stopped doing them.

CHAPTER SIXTEEN

Primary Gain

Tell us your phobias and we will tell you what you are afraid of.
— Robert Benchley

I had been invited to be the visiting professor at neurology Grand Rounds at one of the other medical schools in Chicago. Neurology Grand Rounds are pretty much the same no matter which medical school is involved. The proceedings start with the presentation of an interesting patient. If there's a visiting fireman, the patient invariably has one of those diseases in which the visitor specializes. This is as it should be; the object of the exercise is education, and the reason for inviting a guest expert is so that he can share his particular expertise. The patient is presented and discussed, with the guest acting as the main discussant. This is then followed by a formal lecture by the guest. I was going to talk on "Recent Advances in the Treatment of Parkinson's Disease." Since they undoubtedly would want to avoid repetition, I was fairly certain that the patient would not have Parkinson's disease. He or she would more likely have some other movement disorder for me to discuss. But which one? Huntington's chorea? Tardive dyskinesia? Tourette's syndrome? Or perhaps some sort of dystonia. The dystonias are a group of neurological disorders that cause abnormal movements that are characterized by sustained postures unlike more rapid, briefer movements that are typical of other movement disorders. All things come and go. Recently there had been an increased interest in the dystonias. Wherever I went, they showed me a patient with dystonia. Why should today be any different? No reason at all.

I sat in the front row as expected, but way over to one side. That way I could watch the audience as they watched the patient, listened to the history, asked their questions, and listened to my questions and comments, and thereby judge their understanding and responses. As I looked around, I realized that, aside from three people, it was an audience of strangers made up of medical students and residents and faculty. The exceptions were the chairman of the department, whom I had known since he became part of the Chicago neurological scene ten years earlier, one of the other senior neurologists, and one of the residents. The latter had been one of the students I had taught at Rush two years earlier. She had been a very good student, bright, hardworking, conscientious, and serious. Too serious, perhaps. Her countenance always bordered on the stern. And she was quiet. Not just soft-spoken, but quiet. She manifested a reticence that bordered on withdrawal. Her presentations had been crisp, lean, spare, all but telegraphic. Not that she omitted anything that was significant; for as far as I knew, she never had. But she never added anything that was peripheral or tangential. None of the gossipy tidbits that make a patient come alive or any of those self-propagated responses that tell more about the presenter than the patient. Her delivery had been dry and impersonal.

She looked toward me.

I smiled at her. I had not known that she was a resident here. I had not even known that she had gone into neurology.

She nodded back. A polite nod. Nothing more.

It was time to start. The senior resident got up on the stage, made a few announcements, introduced me, and then began to relate the patient's history. The patient was a twenty-eight-year-old bisexual intravenous drug user.

The cat was out of the bag. The differential diagnosis of neurological disease in a twenty-eight-year-old bisexual intravenous drug abuser has in the last few years become fairly short. It's not that a wide variety of diseases no longer occur in such individuals. They still do. As far as I know, there is no neurological disease that being bisexual protects against. Nor being an intravenous drug abuser for that matter. But being either shifts the odds away from anything else toward AIDS and its diverse complications. Markedly shifts.

The patient was known to have AIDS, the resident announced.

Completely shifts.

His AIDS had been initially diagnosed in New York, at Bellevue, following an episode of pneumonia.

"Pneumocystis carinii?" someone from the audience asked.

Yes. The patient had been treated for that twice. Once in New York. And once in L.A., at L.A. County. They had sent for the records, but the patient had been in the hospital for only two days. It usually took four to six weeks to get the records from L.A. County, and from New York, months.

He had also been treated at Cook County and at a couple of private hospitals in the Chicago area. His family was from Chicago. He had come home to live out whatever remained of his life with his family.

He had come home to die, I thought to myself.

And he was only twenty-eight. Around the same age as the residents. An embarrassed, uncomfortable hush fell over the room. Every judgment that had been made on the basis of the original description of the patient as an IV drug abuser was now a cause for guilt and regret.

But what, I wondered, was the neurological problem?

That had started about one year earlier, while Mr. Kline was living in L.A. He had been at a party. He was a guitarist who had worked with various bands and groups in New York and L.A. He had even made records. The senior resident then listed a number of rock groups with which the patient had played. I had never heard of any of them, but the twenty-eight-year-olds in the audience obviously had. There was a buzz. Excitement. And something more. I wasn't certain exactly what.

I looked around the room. Sadness was reflected on virtually every face. All save one. My old student. Her expression had not changed. As usual, she reflected no emotion. No response. No editorializing whatsoever.

Mr. Kline had been playing his guitar at the party and had been sitting cross-legged on the floor for about two hours. When he tried to get up his left knee would not bend. Or more accurately, it would not unbend. It remained frozen in place. His friends took him to L.A. County. He was admitted to the orthopedic service. They were sure he had something in his knee joint, a torn piece of cartilage that had become dislodged, had floated into the wrong spot and wedged in there, and was preventing his knee from bending.

The next day, he underwent orthoscopic surgery. And postoperatively, his knee was straight. Now, however, he couldn't bend it. It stayed like that for two weeks.

The orthopedic surgeons repeated the orthoscopic surgery. Following the second procedure, Mr. Kline's knee was bent just as it had been prior to the first exploration. The orthopedic surgeons had no idea what to do. There had been no fragments in the knee joints. They called in neurology to see if there was some neurological explanation for his abnormal postures. The next day a neurologist came to see him.

Who? I wondered. There were no well-recognized experts on movement disorders in L.A. Still, he didn't need an expert. The diagnosis was fairly clear.

The neurologist made a diagnosis of dystonia.

Everyone in the audience nodded appreciatively. In their minds, it was a good diagnosis. And it had been made quickly, far more quickly than it usually was. Most patients with dystonia saw any number of physicians before the correct diagnosis was made. Often more than one neurologist. Here the first neurologist had made the diagnosis of dystonia.

The term dystonia was first used by a German neurologist named Oppenheim, early in this century, to describe a specific hereditary disease characterized by abnormal (dys) muscle tone (tonia) and peculiar abnormal movements. We now apply his word as a descriptive term to a class of abnormal, involuntary movements. Dystonic movements are abnormal movements that are rather slow, neither brief, sudden jerks or twitches, or rhythmic tremors. And dystonic movements always produce abnormal postures or positions of the involved part of the body. And this posture lasts for at least seconds.

Frank Kline had been diagnosed as having dystonic movements. But what was the cause of the movements? Dystonic movements can be seen as part of the slowly progressive hereditary disease originally described by Oppenheim. Clearly, Frank Kline did not have a slowly progressive hereditary disease.

He had AIDS.

We all knew that. His doctors in L.A. knew that. His AIDS had been diagnosed in New York the year before.

Dystonic movement can also be caused by any number of diseases of the brain if they cause injury to those deep regions that control movement — the basal ganglia, especially one particular basal ganglion called the putamen.

The neurologist at L.A. County had reached the same conclusion. Kline had to have an infection of the brain, an infection involving the putamen. In all probability, he had some opportunistic infection that had started up because he had AIDS and could not combat infections normally. They were certain he had an abscess. The only question was what caused the abscess.

Toxoplasmosis?

Or cryptococcosis?

It could be any one of those rare infections that occur only in patients whose immune systems have failed. In patients with AIDS.

A diagnosis of toxoplasmosis had been made. Frank had been treated appropriately, and he had made a complete recovery.

Everyone in the audience was pleased. Pleased and proud. The neurologists had come through. The orthopedic surgeons had had no idea what was wrong. Neurology triumphant. What could be better at a neurology Grand Rounds?

It was to be a short-lived triumph.

Frank had moved back to Chicago. The prognosis for AIDS, once brain infections set in, is not good, even if the first one responds well to treatment.

Frank did well for the next six months.

The transition was not lost on me. From anonymous twenty-eight-year-old bisexual, intravenous drug abuser, to AIDS patient, to Mr. Frank Kline, to Frank. From case to friend. Soon there would not be a dry eye in the house. Except Joanne Mitchell's, I said to myself, finally recalling her name. Mine were also dry.

Six months ago, it had happened again. He had had a second episode of the sudden onset of dystonia. This time his dystonia involved his right leg, which became bent and frozen in place.

He was taken to a suburban hospital. There he was seen by

another neurologist, who made the same diagnosis that had been made in L.A.: dystonia due to an abscess in a patient with known AIDS.

The question was once again the same. What kind of abscess did he have?

They made a diagnosis of toxoplasmosis and treated him successfully.

Another triumph. Once again, Frank was discharged from the hospital. But not for long. Soon he developed another episode of pneumonia. This time he was treated at Cook County Hospital.

Home again. Only to have more problems. Weight loss. Fevers. Dystonia of the left leg, with his knee bent back 120 degrees and absolutely immobile.

Another hospital.

Another neurologist.

Same diagnosis.

Same treatment.

Another success, of sorts.

And then, two days before this admission, his dystonia had started again, in the left leg. One minute Frank's leg had been fine, the next, severely deformed. Bent. Frozen. Immobile. Dystonic.

They wheeled him in on a stretcher. He was flat on his stomach. He was thin. And wasted. Malnourished. With his left leg bent at the knee, 120 degrees at least.

I was asked to examine him.

I did.

His knee was as advertised. Frozen. Immobile. I could not move it.

End of examination. I sat back down. Everyone seemed dissatisfied. Including both Frank Kline and Joanne Mitchell. But I had done all I had to do.

Others in the audience asked him questions. Especially the chairman, Bill Baumeister. "Frank," he began, "tell us about your dystonia."

Frank did. From the beginning. Each episode had been the same. Each had started suddenly, like a bolt out of the blue.

"How suddenly?" I interrupted.

"Immediate. One second I was okay. The next second it was there," the patient told me.

"Did it get worse?"

"No. Each time it starts as bad as it can be."

That meant that there had been no progression. He had had the acute onset of abnormal posture that never got any worse. Once the neurologists made the diagnosis and treated him, he got better.

"How?" I asked.

Frank didn't understand.

"Quickly? Or slowly? Did it go away quickly, all of a sudden, or slowly?"

"All of a sudden."

He talked a lot more. About the pain. The immobility. I asked no more questions. They wheeled him out.

Baumeister asked me to go up on the stage and talk about Mr. Kline's disease, since it was one of the newest problems facing neurology, the neurological complications of AIDS. I could, of course, focus on my special area of interest, abnormal involuntary movements related to AIDS and its complications.

I could feel the excited anticipation. This was the first patient they had ever seen with this problem, and here was the expert.

"The patient," I began, intentionally not calling him "Mr. Kline" and certainly not "Frank," "has one of the oldest problems in neurology, the problem of whether or not a patient with a set of signs and symptoms has any neurological disease at all."

The audience buzzed.

"As far as I can tell, Mr. Kline does not."

Excitement changed to surprise.

"And he certainly does not have dystonia."

And surprise to dismay.

To anger.

Not at Frank Kline, but are Harold Klawans. Some expert!

"How can you say he doesn't have dystonia?" Baumeister challenged me.

I reminded them of the definition of dystonia — an abnormal involuntary movement that maintained an abnormal posture for seconds.

Not minutes.

Not hours.

Not days.

And certainly not weeks.

Seconds.

I reminded them of the other characteristics of dystonia. Torsion. Twisting. The movement always has a rotary or torsion component. For years it was called torsion dystonia.

Mr. Kline had no component of torsion. None at all. Just flexion at the knee.

And his movement had started suddenly and had immediately reached its maximal degree. I'd never seen that in any patient with any kind of dystonia. Had anyone else?

No one said anything.

I had never read about such a patient. And I was fairly sure I had read most of the world's literature on dystonia. I'd never read of such a patient. Not in English. Or German. Or French. Had anyone else?

Silence greeted my question. An angry silence. I may have been convincing them, but I wasn't winning any friends.

Dystonia, I admitted, was a clinical diagnosis, and I couldn't prove that he didn't have it. There were no tests for dystonia. But Frank Kline did not have dystonia.

"Why would Frank invent such a symptom?" someone asked.

That I couldn't say. At that point, a psychiatrist got up and talked about hysteria and the deep-seated neurotic needs of patients with hysteria. The audience listened sympathetically. Poor Frank had AIDS and deep-seated psychiatric problems too. That was why he had turned to drugs in the first place.

"Secondary gain," someone else suggested. "He had to do it to get our attention and the kind of medical care he deserves. None of us really give AIDS patients the help they deserve."

I was in no mood for such guilt trips.

"Be careful about that term secondary gain," I said. And I told them about primary gain. Traditional psychiatrists focus on secondary gain, the secondary advantage a patient derives from an illness, but not related to the primary, psychiatric reason for developing the disease. What is often overlooked is primary gain. I told them the classic story of the soldier in the front line in the Korean War. His best friend gets killed. Blown to bits in front of him. The soldier reaches out and touches the body. Or what is left of it. Suddenly, he can no longer move his hand.

Hysterical paralysis.

Classic Freudian conversion hysteria.

Why?

Because of some deep-seated neurotic conflict? That would be the classic analytic interpretation.

I didn't accept that.

His secondary gain? To get attention? Love?

Hell no.

Life did not require such convoluted interpretation. He was interested in a primary gain. He wanted to get the hell out of there and not get killed. An admirable motivation.

Now I could feel their anger.

Was I saying that Frank was malingering? That he was faking his dystonia?

He did not, I reminded them, have dystonia.

If they had had tomatoes, they would have thrown them at me. I was glad they didn't. And even happier they didn't have stones.

"And why, Professor Klawans," Baumeister said, standing up, "would a patient dying of AIDS invent symptoms?"

"I don't even know that he has AIDS."

That was the last straw. I could feel the stones coming my way.

"Nor do you. You did no tests. You took his word for it. The word of a man whose only symptom, I remind you, is entirely factitious."

Abject hatred.

Joanne Mitchell got up. "Dr. Klawans is right," she said.

Everyone turned to face her.

"He does not have AIDS. I was his intern when he was admitted to Sisters of Mercy, four months ago. We treated him for toxoplasmosis of the brain. But all his tests were negative."

The audience was becoming conflicted, ambivalent.

"We sent for his records. They came after he was discharged.

L.A. County had never made a diagnosis of AIDS. His tests had all been normal. The same thing had happened in New York. As far as we could discover, he had never had pneumonia.

"After he was discharged, the police came by to talk to us. He's wanted in New York on a narcotics charge. He was a big-time pusher. According to them, every time he had a hearing for extradition, he ended up in the hospital."

She sat down.

I was vindicated.

We now all knew about his primary gain. Not as admirable as not getting killed in a war, but just as primary.

The next day I got a call from a police detective. Could I help them? They had all of Frank Kline's records. Could I review them and tell them whether or not he had AIDS? And if he didn't, could I tell them whether he was well enough to travel to New York?

I would be happy to do that, I said.

I never did. By then, Frank Kline had signed out of the hospital and left Chicago. No one knew where he went. And they couldn't ask his family. He had no family. At least not any in the Chicago area.

CHAPTER SEVENTEEN

As Pure as the Driven Snow

"Why did you come to Casablanca?" Colonel Strasser asked.
"I came for the waters," Rick replied.
"There are no waters."
"I was misinformed."

> — From the movie *Casablanca.*

There are a lot of mediocre judges and lawyers
and they are entitled to a little representation.

> — Senator Roman L. Hruska, *in defense of*
> *one of President Richard M. Nixon's*
> *nominees to the Supreme Court.*

Lead poisoning is not a new disease. Lead has been used by civilized man throughout recorded history. The symptoms of lead poisoning were described by ancient European physicians: Hippocrates, Galen, Celsus, to name just a few. But our understanding of the effects of lead exposure has undergone a remarkable evolution in the last few decades. This evolution, like many others, has spawned a number of lawsuits. Purity Hatcher was the plaintiff in one of these suits.

The ancients thought of lead poisoning as a severe disease that began suddenly and was frequently fatal. It was considered to be similar to most such acute disorders. If the patient survived, he returned to normal. That, too, was how we thought about it until 1943. In that year, two American pediatricians named Byers and Lord investigated the late effects of acute lead poisoning.

They studied some twenty children, all of whom had survived episodes of mild to moderate lead poisoning during infancy. All but one of the children were found to be failing in school. Nineteen out of twenty! That meant that it wasn't like pneumonia. People, or children at least, who survived the acute illness often did not make a total and complete recovery. In children, severe lead poisoning usually presents as headache, vomiting, and delirium that progresses to a coma. The children may well recover, but not completely. They look healthy. The headaches disappear. So does the vomiting. They are no longer confused or delirious, but as Byers and Lord discovered, they often do not return to a normal level of mental function.

Why not?

Lead exerts its toxicity by blocking the normal activities of the enzymes of the brain cells. This can result in the death of these neurons. This is especially true during early childhood, when brain cells are particularly susceptible to such insults. It is quite easy to imagine nonfatal lead poisoning killing just enough brain cells to result in permanent injury.

In their pivotal paper, Byers and Lord did more than just document the permanent nature of the brain injury caused by lead poisoning; they also showed that even children with few, if any, obvious signs of lead poisoning could suffer permanent damage. Over the last forty years other investigators have refined our understanding of this process. It is now clear that normal-appearing children with moderate elevations of blood and brain lead levels, not sufficient to cause classical lead poisoning with vomiting, headache, and so forth, also function at a lower level intellectually than children who have lower lead levels. This is an entirely new class of lead poisoning.

But how do kids get lead poisoning?

From the air they breathe and the "food" they eat. Air is not so much of a problem today. The use of lead-free gas has markedly reduced the amount of lead children (and adults) inhale. "Food" remains the big source. Not food, per se, but all of the other things that little kids put in their mouths. At one time toys were a significant source. Toys used to be covered with lead-based paints.

No more. Boys used to play with lead soldiers. No more. Wall paint was also a common source. The paints used in homes used to be lead based. Ingestion of such paints often caused lead poisoning. These paints have long been illegal in the U.S. It has been known for almost two hundred years that the ingestion of such paints causes lead poisoning. It has also been known forever that kids tend to eat flakes of paint and God knows what else. There is even a word for this phenomenon: pica, the Latin word for magpie, now used in medicine to describe the ingestion of nonfood substances, especially by young children.

Purity Hatcher had had lead poisoning when she was only three years old. She had gotten it as a result of pica. She had eaten paint in the building where she lived. And that paint contained lead. I became involved with Purity Hatcher because she (or, more correctly, her mother) had sued the owner of the apartment building in which they lived. It was his paint that Purity had ingested. And it was his obligation to make certain that his building did not present that sort of hazard to children. That's the law in Chicago.

It all began with a phone call from her lawyer, a man named Phil Mulroy. He explained that he had a client with lead poisoning. The lead poisoning had been documented by the Chicago Board of Health. They had treated the child for lead poisoning at age three. The source of the lead was known. The city inspectors had found flaking paint in the common areas of the apartment building — the stair wells, the window frames, the doors, and door frames. The flaking paint contained lead. That flaking paint should have been removed, but never had been. That made the case pretty cut-and-dried. The source of the lead was known. And the occurrence of the disease had been documented.

"Why do you need me?" I asked.

"To prove causation," he said. "For that, I need an expert."

That sounded reasonable. That's how the game is played. Someone has to prove that the lead caused the damage.

"Why me?"

"Frank Larry recommends you very highly."

Frank was a malpractice lawyer and one of my closest friends. If

Frank had recommended me to Mulroy, that meant Mulroy was okay.

"Fine," I said. "Send me the Board of Health records and then I'll examine her."

And in due course, that happened. I received the records of the Board of Health. There was no evidence of any episode of classic lead poisoning. There were just nurses' notes that Purity seemed well. That didn't matter; a child can seem perfectly well and still have brain damage from lead poisoning. It happened every day. The Board of Health had done routine screening for lead poisoning. Purity's blood levels were elevated: 37, 41, 44, 47. Those levels were high enough to cause brain damage. Studies had shown that kids with lead levels above 40 during infancy later have lower I.Q.'s and worse school performance than kids whose levels never went above 30.

So, Purity had had lead poisoning.

And the Board of Health had treated her for it. They had given her shots of EDTA. EDTA is a chelating agent. It is a molecule that has a high affinity for lead. When given, it leaches the lead out of the body. The lead attaches to the EDTA and is cleared from the body in the urine.

After EDTA Purity's urine lead went up and her blood lead level went down. All the way to 10.

Then it went back up.

Why?

She had still been only three years old. She still lived in the same place. The lead paint was still there. EDTA may cure lead poisoning, but it doesn't cure pica. Only normal growth and development does that.

Her level got back to 22. Then 35. But no higher.

At age four, it was down to 28.

At age five, 21.

No more pica.

No more screening.

Her mother brought her in to see me. She told me that Purity had eaten lead paint at their apartment on York Street.

"Did her behavior change?" I asked.

"Yes."

The Board of Health records hadn't mentioned any changes in Purity's behavior, but that didn't surprise me. The notes were put down by nurses working at a frantic pace in an overcrowded clinic. The nurses were hurried. So were the patients. And often it had been the grandmother who had brought Purity to the clinic. And each time it had been a different nurse. No rapport. No patient-doctor relationship. And Mrs. Hatcher had had time to reflect. Two whole years.

What had the changes been?

Purity became less active. She cried more, she would just sit and rock and cry. She did that a lot. And she learned more slowly.

Then the Board of Health treated her with the shots, the EDTA. And things got better. Purity became more active. But she still wasn't a good learner. She was in kindergarten and the teacher had told the mother that her attention was low and that she was a slow learner.

The major question left to answer was whether there was any other potential cause of altered intellectual function. After all, lead poisoning was not the only possible cause. So I asked the mother the important questions. I learned that Purity was the third of three children, that the pregnancy had been normal, and that Mrs. Hatcher had had no illnesses during the pregnancy.

Had she taken any medications during the pregnancy? Just iron and vitamins. Any alcohol? No. Any drugs? No.

The labor had been normal. So had the delivery. She and Purity had gone home on the third day after the delivery.

Purity's development had been just like that of Mrs. Hatcher's other two kids. Maybe faster. Purity walked at nine months, talked at twelve months, and was toilet trained long before she was two.

That meant that pregnancy, labor, birth, and development had all been normal. So there was no other obvious cause for any mental changes.

The examination, itself, was normal. I expected it to be. She looked and acted healthy. Her gross brain function was fine. It would be the subtle aspects of higher brain function that had been injured:

Concentration.

Attention.

Perception.

Intellect.

I called Mulroy. "She had lead poisoning," I said, letting him in on nothing new.

"Did she have any permanent injury?"

Legally, permanency was what would be worth real money.

"The mother says so."

"Terrific."

"But we'll need documentation. She'll need a good evaluation by a trained neuropsychiatrist. A full-scale I.Q. Tests of perception, attention, all that."

"When?"

"Before I testify to any permanence."

"They're going to settle."

"I also need all the other records."

"What other records?"

"Birth. Delivery."

"All normal."

"I'll need to see them, just the same."

"No problem."

Two weeks later, he called back. The defendants wanted to settle but he needed a letter saying that Purity had lead poisoning.

"I can't prove the degree of damage yet," I said. "The permanence. I need the testing."

"They want out. Send me a report."

I did. The report was short. It said exactly what I could say and pointed out precisely what I could not say. I wrote that it was my opinion, based upon my review of the history I had obtained from the mother, my review of the Chicago Board of Health records, and my own detailed neurological examination, that Purity Hatcher suffered from lead poisoning. Further, this episode had occurred while she was living in an apartment on York Street and her lead poisoning had required treatment by the Board of Health. I also wrote that at the time of this exposure, there was a history of a change in personality. According to the mother, she became less alert and less active. The mother reports that subsequently Purity has been slow in acquiring and learning new information.

In essence then, I told them that Purity had had an episode of lead poisoning and had a history of learning deficits that were consistent with that history. I pointed out that further psychometric evaluations would be helpful in defining the extent of these deficits.

And that was that.

Until four years later when I got a phone call from Phil Mulroy. I did not remember him. He told me he had called about a case.

What case?

Purity Hatcher.

I had all I could do to remember her. I pulled out my file.

I thought that that had been settled, I told him.

It hadn't been. And the defense now wanted to take my deposition.

That was no problem, but I needed the records in order to prepare my testimony.

"What records?"

"Board of Health, school, any psychometric testing, birth. All the significant records."

"I'll send you whatever I have."

Two days later we met in his office right before my deposition. He had wanted us to spend an hour and a half to go over my testimony. Lawyers all feel they need that much time. And perhaps with other experts they do. I never allow more than half an hour and I start the discussion by telling them exactly what I can say and what I can't say.

"I can't say any more than I did in my letter. She had lead intoxication. That's not surprising. It's documented by the Board of Health records. They treated her for it. Her mother gives a history consistent with lead poisoning, but you never got the psychometric testing, so I can't describe any permanent damage. None at all. She's an average student, according to the school records. I can give you causation, but damages are a problem. So is permanence."

"Then there's no case."

"That's not my problem. Four years ago I told you to have formal psychometric testing done. Did you ever do that?"

"Not yet."

"The most I can say is that she had lead poisoning and that the level of lead poisoning was sufficient to cause permanent injury. And that further testing is needed to define that injury."

"That's all? It would be better if . . ."

"Better," I interrupted, "it will only be when I get the necessary testing results."

He shrugged his shoulders and sat back. He wanted to tell me what else I shouldn't say.

All I wanted to know was the name and style of the opposing attorney. He was the one who was going to ask all the questions. He was a young lawyer named Coleman from the law firm of Bauer, Mapes, Woodling and Lindell.

I knew the firm. I had worked for them in the past. Not for Coleman, but for a couple of the partners. In fact, I was an expert for them in a case that was still going on. That made it unlikely that Coleman would try to attack me.

End of conference.

We then walked over to the offices of Bauer, Mapes, Woodling and Lindell. The court reporter and Joseph Coleman were waiting for us in one of the conference rooms. The offices were on the thirty-seventh floor. And the conference room faced the skyline of the city, north of the Chicago River. The view was spectacular. It contained all the elements that make the Chicago skyline so interesting, modern blocks of steel and glass intermixed with early twentieth-century Gothic stonework, as well as old buildings with water towers. It was a panoramic history of architecture of the last century. All in one glance, on a bright, clear, sunny June day.

The perfect setting for an ambush.

Coleman introduced himself and went to work. First, he reviewed my curriculum vitae with me, starting with my undergraduate education and going on through medical school and residency.

Was I board certified?

I was.

He asked about my publications and my presentations at scientific meetings.

All that certainly qualified me as an expert on neurological diseases.

Did any of those books or papers deal with lead poisoning?

One in particular.

Which one?

Volume 36 of the *Handbook of Clinical Neurology*, of which I was one of the editors. The first three chapters had to do with lead poisoning.

So much for background.

What records had I reviewed?

Board of Health, school, building inspectors.

Had I examined the patient?

I had.

How many times?

Once. Four years ago.

And not since?

Not since.

Had I prepared a report?

I had.

He had a copy. He read it to me. Did I still hold those same opinions?

Yes.

We then went over my opinions in detail.

It was a piece of cake. I stared out the window and tried to guess the decade in which the various rooftops had been built.

Purity Hatcher had had an episode of lead poisoning.

When?

1978.

What was my basis for that opinion?

The records of the Board of Health.

Did those document lead poisoning?

They did.

What was her highest lead level?

Forty-seven. I had done my homework.

Any other basis?

The history given by the mother.

Was that corroborated by the Board of Health records?

No. He, too, had done his homework.

Why was that?

I had no idea. I wasn't there but I had seen that before. The histories obtained in such clinics were often less than optimal.

What was the source of the lead poisoning?

Pica. The ingestion of paint from the apartment on York.

What was the basis of that opinion?

It was, I replied, based on three separate factors: The first was the presence of lead in the paint in various areas of the building as reported by the building inspectors. The second was the well-known fact that the consumption of lead paint was a common, well-documented cause of lead poisoning. Lead paint poisoning had first been described in Australian children toward the end of the nineteenth century. The third was that the child, herself, had been known to ingest the paint.

Who told me that?

Her mother.

Was that documented in the Board of Health records?

No.

Was Purity permanently injured?

"She had had sufficient exposure to lead," I said, "to cause permanent injury."

The basis of that opinion?

I stopped gazing out the window and looked directly at Joseph Coleman. He had a boyish complexion and a slight smile. Ever so slight.

I went over the data from the medical literature, starting in 1943 and the work of Byers and Lord and going up to the far more recent work, especially the study of Perino and Ernhart. They had studied preschool children. Purity had been a preschool child in 1978. Perino and Ernhart had studied children without any symptoms at all. The children had lead levels between 40 and 70. Purity's level had been in that range, 47. That was why the discrepancy between the mother's history and that recorded by the Board of Health nurses was irrelevant. The children studied by Perino and Ernhart were all asymptomatic. They had no symptoms at all of lead poisoning. They compared these thirty children with thirty other children with lead levels below 30. The group with higher lead levels had lower levels of intellectual function.

Did Purity have a decreased level of intellectual function?

I wasn't certain. Her mother gave a history of that but I needed to see detailed testing.

He nodded. Still smiling.

I went back to gazing out the window. A helicopter was crossing the skyline from north to south. I watched it.

"Could other factors affect a child's intellectual function?" he went on.

"Of course."

"Such as?"

"Heredity."

I paused.

Coleman said nothing.

I went on. "Pregnancy."

"What do you mean by that?"

"The fetus is susceptible to any number of things that can happen during pregnancy and cause brain injury."

"Such as?"

"Infection."

"Did Purity's mother have any infections during her pregnancy?"

"No."

"And how do you know that?"

I stopped following the flight of the helicopter.

"I asked the mother."

"Did you ever see her prenatal records?"

"No."

"What else?"

"Other illnesses during pregnancy."

"Was there any evidence of any other illness during pregnancy?"

"No."

"And how do you know that?"

I stopped looking out the window altogether. "I asked the mother."

"Did you ever see the prenatal record?"

"No."

"Anything else?"

"Drugs or medications taken during pregnancy."

"Did Purity's mother take any drugs or medications during pregnancy?"

"No."

And how did I know that?

I was studying Joseph Coleman's boyish face. His expression hadn't changed a bit. He still had a slight smile. Slight but definite.

I had asked the mother.

Had I seen the records?

"That's already been asked and answered," Mulroy said, voicing his objection. "The doctor doesn't have to answer the same question over and over again."

I had forgotten that Mulroy was there. I answered the question. I had not seen her prenatal records.

"Any other factors?"

"Labor."

"Had that been normal?"

"Yes."

My source of that?

Her mother.

Had I seen the labor records?

No.

It had become a routine. He asked me a variety of questions about labor and delivery.

Each time my only source had been the mother. Each time I said I had never seen the records. Each time Phil Mulroy objected. The question about records had been asked and answered. It became a litany. A boring litany. Even Joseph Coleman seemed uninterested. He was reading his questions from a pad of yellow legal paper.

One after another, one fact at a time. Each one followed by the same pair of questions. How did I know that? Had I seen the records?

Then came Mulroy's objection.

Followed by my answer.

Then Coleman asked a different question. Had I requested the records?

"I asked for all significant records, including her birth records."

"You never saw them?"

"Objection. Asked and answered."

"No."

"Let's go back to the pregnancy. You are a pharmacologist as well as a neurologist, aren't you?"

"Yes."

"A professor of both?"

"Yes."

"Tell me, Professor Klawans, what drugs taken during pregnancy can affect the brain?"

"The list is very long. Sedatives, anticonvulsants . . ."

"Maybe it would be better," he said, "if I suggest a few."

"That might be better," I replied. Or it might not. His smile was broadening. He was no longer looking at his list of questions.

"Heroin?" he asked.

I looked at Mulroy. He shrugged and said nothing.

"Possibly."

"Talwin?"

"Possibly."

"Darvon?"

"Possibly."

"Cocaine?"

"Possibly."

"Why are you just saying possibly? Isn't it probable that these drugs taken during pregnancy cause effects on the brain of the child?"

"That would depend on the amount," I replied.

"I object to this entire line of questioning," Mulroy said. "There is no evidence that Purity's mother took any of these drugs at all during pregnancy. She denied such allegations both in talking to this doctor and under oath at her deposition."

"Would you like to know the amount?"

"Objection." Mulroy was shaking his head. "Doctor. You don't have to answer these questions."

By now I was looking directly at Joseph Coleman. His smile was gone.

"Yes."

"Those birth records which you never saw might be very helpful."

"Objection."

"Yes."

"If Purity's mother was a heroin addict who took heroin, Talwin, Darvon, and cocaine during pregnancy, and Purity was born prematurely, would that change your opinion?"

"Objection."

"It certainly might."

"There is no evidence at all of any of this," Mulroy argued. "I can't advise you not to answer a question, Doctor, but . . ."

"Shut up," I said.

"Would you like to see the records?"

"Yes."

He handed them to me.

I read them. They were the medical records of Purity's mother. According to the records, the mother was a known intravenous heroin abuser. She used and abused heroin and Talwin and Darvon and cocaine during the pregnancy. Purity had been born four weeks prematurely.

"Dr. Klawans, now that you've read those records, I'd like to ask you your opinion again."

"I object."

"I'd like that."

"In your opinion, did Purity Hatcher have an episode of lead poisoning?"

"Yes." That had been documented by the Board of Health.

"Did she suffer any permanent injury from that episode?"

"I have no idea at all."

"Why not?"

"Two reasons. There has never been any formal testing. But more importantly, even if there had been, I know of no way to tell whether any permanent deficits would have been caused by the various drug exposures during pregnancy or the lead poisoning at age three."

"You couldn't tell the difference?"

"No."

"Trying to pinpoint one as the major cause would be speculative?"

"Yes. And I don't speculate."

"I'm done," Coleman said.

"So am I," I said.

"I have some questions," Phil Mulroy said, preparing to rehabilitate his case.

"I don't have any more answers," I said. And I got up and left.

As soon as I got to the office, I called Frank Larry. He'd gotten me
into this by recommending me to Mulroy.

I told him what had happened. I had been snookered. I was
angry. My reputation as an expert witness had been sullied.

He doubted that. I had given an honest opinion based on one set
of facts, and when given a second set, had given a second honest
opinion. It happened all the time. No big deal.

"I want to see Mulroy get clobbered."

"Why?"

"Why! Look, there are two possible scenarios. Either he was too
lazy or too incompetent to get those records, or he lied to me.
Either way he ought to be punished."

"He's already been punished."

"How?"

"He lost his case."

"Lost his case. That's not punishment. He never had a case. You
can't lose something that never actually existed."

"But he lost the money," Frank protested.

"Stop talking like a plaintiff's lawyer and think like someone
with ethics."

"Touché."

I took a deep breath. "He lied to me."

"You don't know that for a fact."

"Purity's mother came into my office and gave me a perfect
history of lead poisoning."

"So?"

"She'd never told that to the Board of Health."

"So?"

"Believe me, she never read Volume 36 of the *Handbook of
Clinical Neurology.*"

"Go on."

"And she didn't fail to send me the records, Mulroy did."

"What do you want to do?"

"Lodge a formal complaint. I have to. I was misled. I was lied to. They had no case. If he'd done his homework, he'd have known that. He was either incompetent or devious. In either case, he shouldn't be practicing law."

"Perhaps."

"He deviated from the acceptable standard of care, so to speak."

"That he did. But do you really want to go through with a formal complaint?"

"I know he's a friend of yours."

"I never met him."

"He said you recommended me to him."

"I never did that," Frank informed me. "I never met the man."

I thought back on Mulroy's original words. I told Frank what he had said. He had merely said that Frank had recommended me. Generically. Not specifically to him. But the implication had been there.

"I was misinformed," I said.

"You were."

"I rest my case."

"Come in Monday and we'll draft a formal complaint."

We did.

And Mulroy was slapped on the wrist. Only once. Very lightly. After all, in the minds of the other lawyers who reviewed my complaint, he had already been punished when he lost his case.

AUTHOR'S NOTE

The landmark study by R. K. Byers and E. E. Lord entitled "Late Effects of Lead Poisoning on Mental Development" was published in the *American Journal of the Diseases of Children* (66: 471–494, 1943).

The other study directly referred to is J. Perino and C. B. Ernhart, "The Relation of Subclinical Lead Level to Cognitive and Sensory-Motor Impairment in Black Preschoolers." *Journal of Learning Disabilities* 7: 616–623, 1974.

CHAPTER EIGHTEEN

Double Jeopardy

Surgery is always second-best. If you can do something else,
it's better.

> — Dr. John Kirklin
> *Cardiovascular surgeon*
> *Mayo Clinic*

She got her good looks from her father. He's a plastic surgeon.

> — Groucho Marx

My involvement in the lawsuit was almost as brief and meaningless as my involvement in her care had been. I had been in legal
terms a subsequent treating physician; in other words, I had seen
her in a patient/physician relationship following the event that was
the basis of the lawsuit. I was thus a witness to certain facts — a
witness, not an expert.

It all took place in 1974. Mrs. Bertha Sherman was sixty-four.
She was a widow, her husband having died four years previously.
She had three grown children, a son and a daughter both married
and living in Chicago and another son who lived in California
someplace. He had been married but was now divorced. And there
were a slew of grandchildren. She thought she was in pretty good
health. She knew she smoked far too much (one and a half packs
per day) and had for far too long (forty years, making that a total
of sixty pack-years of smoking) and that because of this she sometimes had trouble breathing and always got short of breath if she
walked too quickly. Her years of smoking had caused permanent
damage to her lungs that obstructed the flow of air in and out. She
had what physicians call COPD, chronic obstructive pulmonary
disease, better known as emphysema.

She knew she had emphysema. She also knew she should quit smoking. And she wanted to stop, but ever since Ralph had died, she just couldn't get up enough energy to do it. And there was no one to help her through the tough spots anymore. If only Ralph were still with her . . .

He, too, had been a smoker. That habit had undoubtedly contributed to his heart disease. Objectively, no one believed that Ralph would have helped Bertha give up smoking. They had smoked together for thirty-six years. Still, it was what she believed. Or wanted to believe.

Her admission to the hospital had nothing to do with her emphysema. She had a small ulcer on her right ear. It was about four millimeters in diameter, but it wouldn't go away. She was admitted so that a plastic surgeon could remove the ulcer and repair her ear. It was no big deal and certainly not a major surgical procedure. Today, it would be done on an outpatient basis. Mrs. Sherman would have been better off if that had been the routine then. But it wasn't.

She was admitted to the plastic surgery service at the hospital. An intern examined her briefly. He noted her history of smoking and shortness of breath. He even wrote down a diagnosis: COPD. And he ordered a chest X ray. The X ray confirmed the diagnosis.

Mrs. Sherman was also seen by an anesthesiologist. He took a history, reviewed her chart, and ordered her preoperative medications. Her surgery was scheduled for 10:00 A.M. Her preoperative medications were to be given "on call to the operating room." That meant that as soon as the operating room called the floor to tell them to send her for surgery, they would give her the preoperative medications the anesthesiologist had ordered.

At 9:15 the next morning, right on schedule, the O.R. called. Mrs. Sherman would be operated on at 10:00 as scheduled.

At 9:20 she got her preoperative medications: Vistaril, a tranquilizer; atropine, to decrease secretions; morphine, for sedation and pain relief.

At 9:30, a man came from transport to take her to the O.R. At that time, transporters were at the bottom of the economic ladder at our hospital, as they were at all hospitals. And still are. Poorly paid. Poorly educated. Poorly trained. And of course, you get what you pay for.

The uniformed transporter picked her up. She was lying on a wheeled stretcher covered by a green blanket and was half-asleep. They began the long, circuitous route to the operating suite. The wait for the elevator was average, about four minutes. And the elevator ride took its usual six minutes, stopping at every floor. The transporter left her outside room six. He even said good-bye. She said nothing. That was not unusual. Doped-up patients often said nothing.

That was at 9:45.

At 9:50 an O.R. nurse came by to take her vital signs and sign her in.

Mrs. Sherman was not breathing.

She hadn't been for several minutes; her lips were blue.

And then, as the nurse was listening, Mrs. Sherman's heart stopped beating.

It was a full-blown cardio-respiratory arrest!

CODE RED!

Controlled panic.

With a flurry of activity.

And a cast of dozens.

Anesthesiologists.

Cardiologists.

Nurses.

CPR.

She responded.

Soon her heart was pounding away. Strong, regular beats.

They stopped breathing for her so that she could start breathing on her own. Nothing happened. No movements of her chest. No air moving in and out.

More artificial respirations.

Another try.

Another failure.

In the end, she was put on a ventilator, which would automatically move air in and out of her lungs.

Her surgery was canceled. And she was admitted to the ICU.

Why had she stopped breathing?

Everyone knew the answer to that question. Someone had screwed up. Morphine and emphysema don't mix well. The respiratory centers of the brain that control breathing are themselves controlled by the blood levels of the two gases, oxygen and carbon dioxide, that are exchanged by the lungs. If the blood oxygen goes down, breathing is stimulated in order to get more oxygen through the lungs and into the blood. In the same way, whenever the blood carbon dioxide goes up, breathing is stimulated, but this time in order to breathe out the excess carbon dioxide. Normally the level of carbon dioxide is the most important factor, and the respiratory center goes along, driven by the blood CO_2 level. In emphysema, this is no longer true. Emphysema is associated with a slow but permanent buildup of blood CO_2 levels. As the blood CO_2 level increases, the respiratory center, instead of continuing to force faster and deeper respiration, adapts to the higher level. Soon, the center no longer responds to any further increases in CO_2, and the only factor left that drives the brain to trigger respiration is the blood oxygen level. Normally that is not a problem, but morphine suppresses the ability of the respiratory center to respond to low oxygen levels. If that occurs, the respiratory center can respond only to increased carbon dioxide. Normally, that is not a problem. But Mrs. Sherman was not normal. She had emphysema. Because of her emphysema, she had been retaining CO_2 for years. Her brain had accommodated to this. Her respiratory centers had become used to it. They only responded to decreased oxygen levels. She was given morphine. Her brain's response to oxygen was suppressed. So she did what was predictable. She stopped breathing.

I saw her two days later in the ICU. The question I was asked was a very simple one. It was the only simple question in her overall medical care. I was asked to determine if she had suffered any brain damage during her arrest. Since she had a tube in her throat that was attached to her ventilator, she couldn't talk to me. She could understand everything I said, and she could write. We conversed for half an hour. She was bright, vital, sharp as a tack. She had a broad range of interests, but soap operas were her passion. She knew everything about them. I knew nothing about the TV soaps, but I remembered the ones I'd heard on radio when I was a child. She also remembered these. We reminisced about them: "Helen Trent"; "Mary Noble, Backstage Wife"; "Portia Faces Life"; "One Man's Family." Enough!

I concluded that there was absolutely no evidence of any brain injury, so I said good-bye and wrote my consult, assuming I would not see her ever again.

I was wrong. She stayed in the ICU. There was no acute problem, but her doctors could not get her off the ventilator. Because of her emphysema, she became adapted to it, and they could not get her to breathe by herself.

The temporary tube was replaced by a permanent tube directly into her trachea by which Mrs. Sherman remained attached to the ventilator.

Each time I went to the ICU to see a consult, she was there.

Day after day.

Week after week.

One month.

Two.

Three.

Four. She became more like an old friend than a patient. Each time I passed her in the ICU she was reading a book, listening to classical music, or knitting. We'd smile at each other, wave, and if I had time, we'd converse about literature or music. I talked. She wrote. She had become a landmark, a permanent part of the hospital landscape: Mrs. Sherman with her ventilator and a new book.

After five months, the plastic surgeon repaired the ulcer on her ear. He did it in the ICU under local anesthesia, without any preanesthetic medication. Just as it would be done today. And should have been done then. But it had been easier to admit her.

Then I heard a rumor that she was suing for malpractice. She probably had a good case. She had emphysema. She should not have been given morphine and then been left without medical supervision.

The anesthesiologist should have known that.

So should the plastic surgeon.

And the intern who wrote her orders.

And the residents who directed her care.

And the nurses who gave her the medicine and then turned her over to a transporter.

Everyone should have known except perhaps the transporter. He had merely transported her. Whether she was breathing or not was an issue that was beyond his competence.

Then one day I was again asked to see her. As soon as I walked into the ICU, I knew something had changed. She was still attached to the ventilator, but she was not sitting up reading.

No book.

No knitting.

No wave.

No smile.

Nothing.

She was now in a coma. In fact, her brain was no longer functioning at all.

She was brain-dead.

What had happened?

No one was certain. All I could tell from the record was that she'd had another arrest.

How?

Why?

When?

It was only the last question that could be answered from the chart. Her arrest had occurred two days earlier.

It was probably a heart attack. Those sixty pack years of smoking had struck again.

I wrote my note. She was taken off the ventilator. That was the end of Bertha Sherman but not the end of the story. The malpractice suit had not been a rumor. She had filed one. And her heirs didn't drop the suit.

Eventually, about two years after her death, I was subpoenaed to give a deposition about what I knew about her care. I knew very little about her overall care. I had seen her only to evaluate her brain function, not to analyze what had caused her respiratory problems.

Prior to my deposition, I met with the hospital's lawyers. They reminded me that I was not an expert witness in this case. I was one of her physicians, a subsequent treating physician. All I had to do was testify about the facts. I was not obligated to give any opinions as to the standard of care. The case, I learned, had become as much a war between the hospital and its lawyers and the physicians and their lawyers as a war between the plaintiff and the defendants. The fact that giving her the morphine was a deviation from the standard of care that had caused her original arrest was uncontested. But who was really at fault?

The plaintiffs didn't care. They'd take money from everybody or anybody.

The hospital put the blame on the anesthesiologist. He should never have ordered the morphine. He had his own malpractice insurance and his own lawyers.

The anesthesiologist blamed the hospital, especially the transporter who worked for the hospital. Had the transporter recognized her respiratory arrest and given her mouth-to-mouth respiration, Mrs. Sherman would never have ended up in the ICU. It was the transporter's fault and therefore the hospital's, since he was a hospital employee.

It was a defense that astounded me. It was like Nixon blaming everything on poor little John Dean. But I had no interest in getting caught in the cross fire, so I decided that I would give no opinions.

The deposition began. The lawyer for the plaintiffs asked the questions. He asked me nothing about Mrs. Sherman's initial arrest or my initial consult or my second consult. He asked only one series of questions.

Did I know what had caused the second arrest?

No.

Did I have any opinions?

What ensued was an all-out war. According to the hospital's lawyers, I was not there as an expert. I wasn't there to give my opinions. The anesthesiologist's lawyer went even further. I was a neurologist. I was not an expert on cardiac arrests. My opinion was worthless. The lawyer for the plastic surgeon agreed but was even more vehement. The plaintiffs' lawyer screamed that he had a right to know the opinions of all subsequent treating physicians as to the medical history.

As I listened to the argument, I began to understand the battle lines. If the second arrest had been a direct result of the first, then, legally, whoever was to blame for the initial event was also responsible for Mrs. Sherman's wrongful death. But if they were unrelated, this would not be true. There would have been no wrongful death unless the second arrest had been caused by another, independent and as yet undefined, deviation from the standard of care. If there had been no malpractice leading to her second arrest, the anesthesiologist would not be at fault for her death. Nor would the hospital. At least not because of the behavior of one of its transporters. Or the plastic surgeon.

A second unrelated act was not what the lawyer for the plaintiffs wanted. A second event that was unrelated to the first meant that he had to prove that the second was a second act of malpractice. It was hard enough to prove one. For if the second was not due to the first and was not malpractice, then it was a result of her own medical condition, and she would have died when she did no matter what. That left the plaintiffs with no wrongful death to be paid for by the defendants. But worse than that it meant that the only damages were Mrs. Sherman's suffering during the five months she was on a ventilator. And how much was that worth? Probably not the $8 million he was asking. After all, even though she was in the ICU, she smiled every day to everyone who came by. And wrote cheerful notes. And read books. And knitted sweaters for the nurses.

He needed that wrongful death.

In the end he asked me his questions.

Everyone put an objection on the record. My answer would count only if the judge overruled all the objections.

Did I have any opinions as to the cause of the arrest?

No.

Had I seen any records describing the exact event?

More arguments.

More objections.

And finally an answer.

No.

End of deposition.

＊　　　＊　　　＊

Six months later the case was settled for around $1 million, one third from the anesthesiologist and two thirds from the hospital. Why had the hospital given so much? I had no idea. As far as I was concerned, the transporter was not twice as responsible as the anesthesiologist.

Two years later I discovered the answer. I learned it from one of the defense lawyers. The hospital knew what had caused the second arrest. They had known all along. Following Mrs. Sherman's first arrest, the hospital decided that the transport service should be upgraded. All transporters were to be trained in CPR. The transporter who had transported Mrs. Sherman was absolutely ineducable. He had no interest in learning. He never made the effort to go to any classes.

The hospital knew that they couldn't fire him. At least not until the case was settled. They changed his job description. He was given a job delivering TV sets to patients' rooms along with flowers and candy and occasional balloons. This way, the most trouble he could cause was to deliver some candy to a wrong room. Or a balloon or two.

No big deal. Nothing that could result in an $8 million lawsuit.

Then one day Mrs. Sherman decided she was bored. She was tired of knitting. She'd read too many books. She'd heard more operas than Toscanini had ever conducted. She wanted a TV set. She wanted to get back to her beloved soaps.

No one in the ICU had ever had a TV set before, but no one else had ever made the request. Every other patient had been too sick. So why not?

There was no reason.

Her doctors ordered her a TV.

Up came the TV. Brought by the same transporter who had delivered Mrs. Sherman to surgery. He walked into the ICU and found the right bed. The patient was napping. There was no reason to wake her up. He'd just plug in the TV, make sure it was working, and take off for lunch. He found the wall sockets. They were all in use. He unplugged the top plug. The bedside lamp went out. He plugged it back in and pulled out the lower plug. Nothing happened. He plugged in the TV, turned it on to *General Hospital*, tuned it in, and left. Mrs. Sherman was reunited with her soaps.

The plug, of course, had been the plug of her ventilator.

Better they should have sent her some flowers. Or balloons.

The suit, I learned, had been settled the day before the transporter had been scheduled to give his deposition.

CHAPTER NINETEEN

Sleeping Beauty

Beware of all enterprises that require new clothes.

— Henry David Thoreau

It was a rainy, cold, windy autumn day in Chicago. Jill Regal was in a hurry. She decided to cut through the new federal office building. It would save her a few steps and, besides, she would be warmer and dryer. She hurried on through, intently watching the slippery floor. As she walked by a row of public telephone booths, one of the wooden doors suddenly flew open and she walked right into it. She was stunned. The door had come out of nowhere.

The frames of her glasses broke.

Her nose began to bleed.

She felt dizzy.

Nauseated.

Light-headed.

She was afraid she would faint.

The floor was so wet.

So slippery.

And she was so dizzy.

So light-headed.

She fainted.

I first saw Jill Regal when I took the stand in federal court as an expert witness in the matter of *Jill Regal v. the People of the United States*. The matter was heard in federal court because the federal government was the defendant. Why was the federal government the defendant?

The accident had occurred in the federal building. The phone booth had been built by the federal government. It was owned by the federal government and had been designed by its architect with a door that opened out into a busy hallway. That was a no-no, a design flaw, architectural malpractice, so to speak.

Whoever had been in that booth had quickly disappeared and could not be found, so there was no codefendant, but the facts of the accident were not being contested. Nor was the error in design. The issue was the damages.

And what were Jill Regal's damages?

According to her lawyer, they were worth a million dollars. But what were they?

A broken pair of glasses, a bloody nose, and one brief fainting spell. Those weren't worth a million bucks.

She also felt sleepy all the time. Tired. Exhausted. Her lawyer's argument was that she had narcolepsy, a serious neurological disorder, characterized by sudden episodes of irresistible sleepiness, that her narcolepsy was totally disabling, and that it had been caused by the head injury. A million dollars was the least she deserved.

I had never examined Ms. Regal, but I had reviewed all of her medical records. As far as I was concerned, she did not have narcolepsy. She merely complained of being fatigued and tired all the time. She had never suddenly gone to sleep. Narcolepsy consists not of feeling sleepy, but of sudden irresistible episodes of sleepiness that cause the patient to go to sleep. There are many causes of being tired. Too many to list. And none is caused by a minor head injury. As far as I could tell from the records, Ms. Regal was depressed. Fatigue and tiredness are common manifestations of depression and after all, she had been hurrying through the federal office building to meet her lawyer in order to discuss her divorce settlement, her husband having run off with a younger woman. And even if she had narcolepsy, as far as I was concerned head trauma did not cause narcolepsy, so the federal government had no responsibility at all for her fatigue.

The trial took place during the summer, and Chicago was in the middle of a heat wave. It was over one hundred degrees Fahrenheit for the sixth straight day. There was no jury. Federal cases are decided by a federal judge, since all jurists as citizens are really, in a sense, defendants in any action against the government.

Since there was no jury, I had no reason to wear my usual conservative testifying suit. Instead, I wore a new red sport coat and a bright pair of striped pants. What could have been more in tune with the season?

Jill Regal's lawyer was not impressed by my outfit. He attacked my opinions as vigorously as he could. I did not cave in. He went over my opinions again and again. I could not be swayed. I stood firm.

She did not have narcolepsy.

And even if she did, trauma did not cause narcolepsy.

Was I certain of that?

I was.

Did everyone else agree with me?

As far as I knew.

All medical authorities?

Yes.

Every one?

Yes.

Was I certain of that?

I was. As far as I knew, no reputable authority believed that trauma caused narcolepsy, and I said as much.

As he got more argumentative, so did I. "No one believes that trauma causes narcolepsy," I declared.

"No one?"

"No one."

"Except for crank lawyers?" he asked.

"No reputable medical authority," I replied.

Weren't there case reports of narcolepsy caused by trauma?

Not as far as I knew.

"None at all?"

"None," I responded, but I was getting a bit wary. He had to be going somewhere.

"So in your expert opinion, there is not a single case report that proves that trauma causes narcolepsy?"

"That's correct."

"And if that case did exist and a reliable authority relied upon it, then you would have to change your opinion."

"Perhaps."

"Certainly you'd have to agree that it has been shown that narcolepsy can be caused by trauma."

"Yes," I conceded grudgingly.

"Are you familiar with the *Textbook of Neurology* by Israel Wechsler?"

I was.

"Isn't it a standard textbook of neurology?"

It was. I didn't like it, but it was widely used. It had been around for years. There had been at least eight or nine editions. I had to agree with him. What else could I do? But what had Wechsler written about narcolepsy?

As I was debating my answer, the lawyer chided me. "Come now, Dr. Klawans. This textbook is already in its fifth edition," he said, lifting up the book. "It must be widely read."

I was certain that it was in its ninth edition, not its fifth. And he had a copy of the fifth. I was no longer worried.

"Yes, I suppose so."

"Well, let me read to you what Dr. Wechsler wrote. 'There are instances in which narcolepsy was caused by head trauma' and he also lists the original case as one of his references." He paused. "So you were wrong, weren't you? There is an authority who believes that trauma causes narcolepsy."

"May I see the book, please?"

He handed it to me. I looked at the cover and then the page from which he had been reading.

"No," I said.

"You are holding the book right in front of you. How can you deny that there are authorities who believe that trauma causes narcolepsy and that there are cases in the medical literature that prove that causal relationship?"

"That's easy. This is the fifth edition of Wechsler's book. That edition was published over thirty years ago. Does Wechsler still believe that trauma causes narcolepsy?" I stared at the lawyer.

He said nothing.

"You don't know. I don't know. Nobody knows. We can't. He's been dead for over a decade. So I still believe that no authority believes, *now* believes, that trauma causes narcolepsy."

"What about the case report?"

"That was published in French in 1906. If that was the only case that Wechsler could find, it certainly doesn't impress me."

Nor did it impress the judge. Jill Regal got a judgment of $900.00.

Two months later, I got a call from her lawyer. He wanted me to act as her expert witness.

Why?

When she'd been taken to the nearest emergency room following her accident, they had given her a shot to quiet her down. He'd done some more reading. That could have caused her narcolepsy.

"But . . ." I tried to interrupt, "she didn't have . . ."

"I have the case reports right here."

I wasn't interested.

Could he send them to me?

"No." And I hung up.

He did file the suit. I don't know who acted as his expert. It wasn't I. It was settled out of court. Not for very much, I hope.

About five years after my role in this case had ended, I happened to run into the judge. He remembered me well. I had won the case for the government. I was impressed that he remembered me. What did he recall? I wondered. My succinct testimony on direct question? My clever response to cross-examination?

"Neither," he said.

"Neither?" I was puzzled. Perhaps it was both. He'd made the decision in favor of the government, and he'd said that I'd won the case. What did he recall? What had swayed him?

"Those pants!" he said.

"My pants?"

"Any expert who had guts enough to testify in pants like that had to be right."

"My pants?" I repeated.

"And that horrible red jacket."